MY LIFE IN A SHORT BUS WORLD

D.A. Perry

Published by BookLocker.com, Inc., St. Petersburg, Florida.

Printed on acid-free paper.

I have tried to recreate events, locales and conversations from my memories of them. In order to maintain their anonymity in some instances I have changed the names of individuals and places, I may have changed some identifying characteristics and details such as physical properties, occupations and places of residence.

BookLocker.com, Inc.
2020

First Edition

This book is dedicated to all the loved ones I lost during while writing this book. I miss you all!

To my step dad Larry you really taught me a lot about being responsible for my own actions in life and showing how a real man acts in the world today

To my grandfather or Papa thank you for always being there for me and for being my first male role model. You are one of the most amazing men I will ever know.

To Daron one of my first real friend's thank you for being a true friend and showing me that my disability wasn't a big deal and my only limitations were in my head.

To Tonya B. I will always consider our friendship a blessing and you were always there when single parenthood got overwhelming or I just needed to hear a calm friendly voice.

Chapter 1

Family is important to me. My mother has been and always will be my driving force. She is the one person that will tell me what I need to hear even if it isn't what I want to hear. My mother also made it very clear to me I can still do anything anyone else can. I just have to want it and work hard for it. I wake up every day with the knowledge that I can do anything,

I was born on December 19, 1970, in Flint, Michigan, the second child of my parents, Diana and Dick. My mom was in labor with me for four days. My disability was very evident at birth. My legs were twisted round and round each other twice, much like a corkscrew. I also had numerous other visible deformities and muscle problems. My mom tells me that I always cried. To change my diaper, she had to untwist my legs and lay on them while she changed me. She also would have to feed me lying down because it was the only way I could swallow. My father was unable to handle my disability. He soon walked out on us and left us with nothing.

Let me paint a picture for you. Here is my mom, 19-years-old, with two kids under the age of 4, one of which was disabled. She had no high school diploma, no real job skills, and worst yet, no health insurance. I doubt anyone would have blamed her if she would have crawled into a hole and never came out. But my mom is an extraordinary lady. She knew she had two kids to support. She couldn't quit. One of the first problems she had to face was that she needed to have me diagnosed. She knew I had medical issues, but she did not know from what or why. She took me to doctor after doctor looking for answers. None of them could give her a straight answer as to what it was and what caused it.

A doctor saw my mom with me and asked her what was wrong. She went on to tell him how she wasn't sure but that she was desperate for answers.

The doctor said to her that he had a few ideas. He wanted her to come for an appointment the next day. My mom said she would but that she was worried because she didn't have health coverage. The doctor said not to worry about that. He just wanted to help her get some answers. The next day, I was looked at by a few doctors, and they diagnosed me with Cerebral Palsy. This disability occurs when there is a loss of oxygen during birth.

The doctor gave my mom a referral to a hospital in Detroit that had a specialist who handled children with Cerebral Palsy by the name of Dr. Maurice Castle at the Neuromuscular Institute. I can tell you right now that they were miracle workers. Without all the work, time, and effort that Dr. Castle did, no way would I have accomplished all that I have today. Once my mom was able to get me diagnosed, she was able to get health coverage under a Crippled Children's program. I still find it hard to believe that none of the other doctors were able to give my mom any answers for the first two years I was alive. One can only imagine the frustration she must have been feeling.

Once my mom was able to get me diagnosed, she went to work on another problem. She knew to care for us; she needed an education. My mom was able to get her high school diploma. But she had bigger dreams. She started college with her aim at an accounting degree. I give my mom a lot of credit for not letting anything stop her. My older sister Kayla and I never really knew all the struggles we faced. Mom made sure that we had what we needed. We had love, and after all, that is the most important thing.

My mom would be the first to tell you that she could not have done it all by herself. My dad left us with nothing, and we had no place to stay. My grandfather bought a trailer and rented it to my mom. When we needed a car or maybe some groceries, my grandparents made sure we had it. Whenever I had an operation, I always stayed with my grandparents. My grandmother would take care of me.

I know life is complicated. It is how you handle those complications and how they affect you that make you who you are. As a child, you learn from your parents and those around you. I was fortunate in the fact that I was born to a mother who had dreams and aspirations. She wasn't about to let anything or anyone stand in her way. I have learned from the women in my life that it's ok to cry. I used the anger to push ahead and move forward. You can't let other people's opinions or stereotypes stop you from what you want. I do more in a day than many doctors thought I would do in a lifetime. I owe my strength I have from my mom and my sister. Truthfully they have shown me the way.

My father was the worst. Dick doesn't deserve to be called anything other than a sperm donor. There is no other way to put it than he abused me almost every way imaginable. I don't believe Dick ever had a kind word to say to me. He made it clear to me that the only reason he left my mother was because of my disability. He was ashamed of me. No matter what I did it was wrong. He yelled at me every chance he got for the things that I couldn't do. I was unable to use the bathroom without assistance until I was five. But in his mind, I should have been able to. He refused to help me. If I was wearing a diaper, he refused to change it the entire time I was with him. Kayla was the only hope I had during our weekends with him. If she didn't help me or change me, I would sit in soiled clothes the entire time.

When he wasn't yelling at me, he would smack me around or spank me. One time I was about four, and we had stopped to get ice cream. I remember it was soft serve with the shell topping on it. I didn't eat it fast enough, and it melted, and I made a mess. Dick beat me in the face and head many times. Kayla was screaming and crying for him to stop. He took me back to my mom and yelled at her because I made a mess. He said I was a waste, and it was all her fault.

With my dad at Christmas time, I remember sitting in the corner with two or three small gifts in front of me. Kayla had a pile. Everyone seemed to be talking to Kayla while they ignored me. They treated me like I wasn't a real human being. I know what some of you are thinking. Why would my mom send me over there? Well, that answer is simple; she had to. The courts made her, and they wouldn't listen to the abuse claims. If she tried to go against the court order and they threatened to throw her in jail. How on earth, a judge could throw a young mother in jail for trying to protect her disabled child is beyond me.

Thankfully Dick eventually moved to Florida. I no longer had to visit him every other weekend. He then refused to pay child support. My mom found out once that he was coming into town for a wedding. She called the police and told them when and where to find him. When they let him out, the first thing he did was to come over to the trailer and break-in. Once inside, he preceded to beat the living hell out of my mom. My lasting memory of Dick is him beating my mother while she tried to protect Kayla and me. I will never forget how bad Dick treated me. And it did leave a lasting effect on my life.

I thought it is important to start talking about my family for many reasons. I felt that you needed a sense of who they were and what they meant to me. I want people to know what motivates me. I agree with the saying that you can't pick your family. I really wouldn't trade mine at all. My family has been with me through the good and the bad times. Not a day goes by that I don't thank God that I have them. They are always there to scoop me up and dust me off. The most important thing I believe for any family members of disabled people to know is you can't treat us any differently. We may need more support. We may also need an extra kick in the butt. You must let them know that they can do whatever they want. They should be encouraged to try anything they want. The first time I tried a lot of things, I failed. My mom always urged me to keep trying.

Chapter 2

The biggest lesson my mom learned about having a disabled child was you have to anticipate unexpected problems. She thought that the biggest challenge was getting me diagnosed to get me medical help. What she learned, however, was that for every challenge, she would solve another issue would then take its place. She knew, however, that I couldn't fight for myself, so she had to be my voice.

Most of the early memories I have as a kid involve hospitals and surgeries. I still, to this day, get the cold sweats when I smell a hospital. My mom always told me she was doing what was best for me. I had a hard time understanding why all this pain was the best thing. She was right, and if she hadn't done that, then no way would I be who I am today.

For many years my life was surgery, then recovery, then another surgery. I had eight surgeries before the age of ten. The first surgery was to uncoil my legs and fix my hips. My hips were being pulled out socket by my muscles. The thing you need to know about Cerebral Palsy is that your muscles work against your body. Your mind says something, but your muscles either do the exact opposite or nothing at all. The first surgery was very complicated and required me to be in a body cast for four months. Now for those of you who have never seen a body cast let me explain. It was a cast that started in the middle of the chest and went to my toes. Another part of the cast had my legs spread as far apart as possible with a bar running between them so that my hips would set in place. The surgery was in two sections. First, they did my left side and then onto the right side. Between the ages of two and three, I was in a cast for eight of the twelve months.

One good thing that happened with the surgery is that I no longer constantly cried. I was able to allow my mother to sleep without strapping me to her. As usual, however, as we solved one problem, another would soon take its place. We would quickly get our first taste of disability discrimination.

When my mom started going to school full time, she needed to find child care. She could not find a daycare that would take me. The state had a rule that a daycare needed one worker per fifteen kids. However, if you had a disabled child there, the ratio then went to one worker per three kids. So if a daycare had sixteen kids and one was disabled, they needed six workers instead of two. My mom had to rely on relatives and babysitters that she hired. She had many problems finding and keeping babysitters. Most could not handle all the special care that I required.

One of the stories she tells is while she was working one night. She got an emergency phone call from a neighbor telling her that she had to get home right away. The babysitter just walked out and left Kayla and me alone. When she got home, there was a letter on the table saying she couldn't take it and she quit. Can you imagine just quitting and leaving two small children home alone at night without warning?

When my mom had school, she talked to her teachers to allow her to bring me to class. I would lay on the floor and color or play with cars. My mom promised them I would be quiet, and I can promise you I was. My mom was very strict. We always knew if she wanted us to be quiet, we better be. To this day, if mom snaps her fingers, my sister and I both stop and look. And if she ever snapped her fingers and stomped her foot, we were dead.

Even though we had apparent financial problems, my mom did what she could to hide it from us. Granted, as a kid, you don't know what poor is. I know now that my mom went without so Kayla and I had what we needed. I remember times when we were eating that she wouldn't eat. I asked her why she would say because she already ate. It wasn't until later when I was much older than she admitted there were many times she didn't eat. She had just enough for Kayla and me to eat. Even thinking about it now makes me want to cry because it proves the level of the sacrifices she made for us.

Our favorite activity was going to the library for story time or sitting together and reading. Little did I know then that the reason we did it was that it was free. I can remember sitting with mom in a giraffe shaped chair and reading books together. The library also had free movies, so we always went to those. My mom would pop our popcorn and put it in small bags for Kayla and me. She would hide it and then give it to the concession lady. She would then give it to us so we would think it was the popcorn the library had. My mom didn't have the extra twenty-five cents for us to buy it there.

Leaving the trailer as a child was not easy for me at all. Back then, they didn't have wheelchairs for children. I still wasn't able to stand, so the only way I could get around inside was by pulling myself with my arms kind of like a military crawl. Even when I had casts on my legs, I would still get around the trailer pretty well. Because of the lack of wheelchairs, my mom usually ended up using an oversized baby stroller that I barely fit in. Our other option at the time was a wagon. My mom or Kayla would prop me up in it and pull me around where ever we had to go.

As I was able to get out more, I got my first taste of bullying. I will be the first to admit that kids can be ruthless. The meanest of them all are the boys. I think it comes from the fact that boys are always trying to prove how tough they are. They do this by picking on the ones they perceive to be the weakest. I was a straightforward target, even at a young age. All I wanted to do was play with the other boys.

The so-called leaders would instead tease me for the way I looked or the way I moved. And the others would join in so that they could fit in with the larger group. I am not going to lie and say that the words or the imitations didn't hurt because they did. The hardest part was trying not to show them that they hurt me. I would get so angry and frustrated. I would start to cry because it seemed to be the only way I could release all the emotions that I had inside.

Bullying was not the only obstacle I would face as my world grew, and I was able to get outside more. When I was young, there weren't even wheelchair, accessible parking spaces. If somewhere did have them, there was no law against parking in them. People would park in them anyway. If you told the police they couldn't or wouldn't do anything about it. One time that I remember around Christmas time, and it was snowing. My mom took us to the mall. She tried to park in a handicapped space. A guy raced into it and parked, then got out and tried to walk away. She stopped him and tried to explain that I was disabled. He admitted he wasn't disabled. He just wanted a close parking space. Then he said he didn't care that I was disabled and wished her a merry Christmas. I thought my mom was going to kill him. My mom found a police officer and told him the story. He said that it wasn't illegal to park there. So she had to park way out and drag me through the snow.

My mom started preparing me to deal with obstacles when she wasn't around. I had to learn very early on how to think outside the box. I think that term is overused, but for me, it is how I live my life. Before I go anywhere or do anything, I have carefully thought out numerous plans if this happens or that happens. So if I do have issues, I can think quickly and not waste time. The only reason I can do that now is that I was raised at an early age to do it then. My mom would ask me many times OK if I wasn't here to help with this what would you do. I would have to answer her, or she would give me options as to what I could have done.

When you have a disabled child or family member, you can't just start pushing them all of a sudden. You have to start slowly with small tasks and simple questions. You have to build up their self-confidence. The more self-confidence they have, the more they can do. You are doing the family member a disservice by not having them do things for themselves. A child with a disability may need more encouragement. You can't ever give up on them because they will give up on themselves. Everyone struggles with something in life. What makes being disabled mainly from birth different is we have struggled from day one.

I was slowly learning how to be independent around the house. Some significant changes were happening to us. My mom bought a small three-bedroom house in Flint, Michigan. The house was a perfect starter home for us. Not long after we moved, my mom started dating a man named Alex. My mom had dated on and off over the years, but Alex was different. He tried to spend time with Kayla and me instead of just dating mom. I did like him from the start because he did his best to be that male influence or father figure that I was missing.

Alex's parents had a lot of money, and we met them not long after they started dating. I remember we drove up to this huge house that looked almost like a mansion that you see on television. Alex's parents seemed nice, although they were not very affectionate. I didn't know what it was at the time, but now I see that they were very snobby. His parents seemed to look down at my mom because she was young and divorced with two kids. Whenever we were around them, we had to act just so. We had to seem to be the perfect family. Mom and Alex got married on a cold December day when I was about nine.

I had dreams of what it would be like to have a dad. Alex had dreams too, but unfortunately, his were not the same as mine. He got in his head that I could do more than I was already doing, and I could do it all his way. I am not against doing anything new to help out around the house. I can't always do things the same way someone wants them done. I think Alex thought that if he pushed me enough or forced me to do things his way that I would automatically do them. Alex never really understood the complexity of my disability. This always seemed like an overwhelming theme with any male influence in my life.

Sadly all the dreams I had as a kid for father-son activities soon died as well. I am a huge sports fan. I am a diehard Wolverine, Tiger, Lion, and Red wing fan. I always dreamed about having the kind of dad that would take me to sporting events. That wasn't Alex. He was into cars, motorcycles, and construction. He could care less who won what game or anything about sports. He was more into fixing his motorcycles or building stuff. They were things that I had no interest in and had no interest in learning. Alex wanted me to be more like him. I wanted him to be more like what my ideal father was.

There were numerous times he would promise to take me to a Tiger game only to come up with excuses after excuse why he couldn't. I acted like it didn't bother me. I have to admit inside it did upset me very much. The one thing Alex did do once in a while he took me to tractor pulls and monster truck shows. They are OK but if you aren't a car guy they can be very dull. I was just happy that I was getting some father-son time regardless of what it was. I guess to me, when you are a father, you need to find things that your child enjoys, not just the things that you like. Parenting to me is as much about sacrifices as anything else.

My mom decided that she wanted to live in a safer area and a better school district. She started looking and houses in Fenton. Before long, she found a home that fit our needs. Going from Flint to Fenton was a lot of culture shock for Kayla and me. I was still going to school in Flint, but Kayla was getting ready to start in Fenton.

I love Fenton; the neighborhood was quiet. We could fall asleep without the sounds of sirens and gunshots. We could go outside without much of a worry. I still didn't go out much once we lived there because I didn't have any friends there. I was still going to school in Flint because Fenton said they didn't have the facilities to handle a student with my disabilities.

After moving to Fenton, Alex decided he wanted to adopt Kayla and me. I was all for this. I would finally have a real dad. I felt like I was putting my birth dad entirely out of my life. Dick called and talked to me about it. This was the first time I had heard from him in years. We had a bizarre conversation. Someone wanted to adopt his kids. They will no longer be his, and instead of being upset, he wasn't. He was happy he wouldn't have to pay my mom child support anymore. Nothing about how much he loved me or he was sorry about everything. It was still all about him and his damn child support.

As the years went by, the marriage slowly fell apart. Alex wasn't a massive fan of working, but he loved to spend money. That led to a lot of fights. When I was about fourteen, my mom had finally had enough and decided to divorce Alex. I can't say I was surprised, but I was still upset. I was angry because Alex was my dad. Divorce on children is complicated. I did blame myself. You always think this would not have happened if I was a better son. My mom did her best to tell me that it wasn't my fault. She was there as much as she could be to try and explain what was going on. Regardless of what my mom said, I still felt partially responsible. I can't even really begin to tell you all the emotions I was going through at the time.

The hardest part of the divorce was my relationship with Alex. One father had already abandoned me. I was scared! I was now on the verge of being left by my second father. Alex did his best at the start saying he would still be there for Kayla and me. He told us that he was our father and had every intention of being one. And in the beginning, Alex did a great job at it. He would pick me up and spend time with me. Alex was doing more with me at the start of the divorce then he ever did while he was married to my mom.

Unfortunately, Alex only picked me up once for a weekend visitation. After that, he would call me with an excuse after excuse. He was busy without a real reason. Then slowly, his calls became less and less. When Alex did call, it was more excuses. Eventually, he was out of my life for good without a word. I struggled for a while because I had been adopted once and abandoned by two different fathers. I was especially struggling in school. I just couldn't focus on my emotions all over the place.

Chapter 3

Early in life, at school was the one place that I felt comfortable. It was the one place there were other kids like me. I looked forward to going to school as a child. I loved the fact when a teacher asked a question, and I usually knew the answer. In school was the first place in the world; I realized I could do more than some kids. Some subjects, especially math, came very easy to me. I could look at problems, and I knew the answer instantly.

The way it worked back then all the schools in the area bussed their disabled children to one school. That school was called Durant Tuuri Mott or as we always called it DTM. I can remember being in shock at first. You think, as a kid, you are the only one in a wheelchair or that is "special." This school had hundreds of kids, most of them with health issues worse than mine. I remember being on a bus with other kids. My mom says I cried a lot when I first started and begged never to go back. But to her credit, she made me go every day.

The school was divided by grade, much like every elementary school is today. You would have kids with differing abilities all in the same room. I could be sitting next to someone with a very severe disability. All they could do was blink their eyes and drool. Even in school, we were very sheltered. The school was in two sections. There were the disabled section and the part of the school for all the kids in the area. And the two sides hardly ever mixed.

I give special education teachers a lot of credit. They may have had only 15-20 kids, but it had to have been hard to come up with lesson plans. They would have needed different lesson plans for each student, depending on their abilities. Besides having regular classes at DTM, each student also had a gym, occupational therapy, physical therapy. They had every kind of treatment that a student may have needed. I think that's why the area schools bussed everyone to that one location. It had to be more cost-effective, having all the help and facilities in one place as opposed to each school spending money on the same thing. I don't think it was a perfect ideal social setting as far as preparing you for the real world.

Making friends for me was never that easy. I was always jealous of Kayla because she could walk to her friends' houses or have sleepovers. I could never do that. My friends all lived a long distance from me. Going to someone else's house wasn't exactly straightforward. All I could do was talk to my friends on the phone, and I did that a lot. My best friend for most of elementary was Billy. I only saw him at school during lunch or on the bus. We always sat and talked about standard stuff or played during recess.

The first few years of school, all I was around were other disabled children, aides, and teachers. You can get very used to being sheltered if that's all you are around. The disabled classes were not challenging me. Between all the therapy and stuff, I don't remember doing much school work. The school only seemed to maintain what I could already do. They were not concerned about teaching new things. I finished most of the work I was given early and just sat there most of the time. I believe it was in second grade where they finally realized my body might be disabled; my mind itself worked just fine.

They started checking into what they called "mainstreaming" me. What that meant was I would still have some classes in the disabled section, but I would also have courses in the regular school as well. They had me take multiple tests to prove myself. I don't remember the tests themselves so much as being in a room doing school work with no windows all day long. I passed the tests. The school decided I would go to a regular class for math.

My biggest problem with math is I can do most of it in my head, but teachers always demanded I show my work. I write slowly, so while I may have had the right answer, a lot of teachers thought I was cheating. They used to call my mom all the time all to claim I was cheating. Once, they even put me in a room by myself with just a math test and a pencil to prove I wasn't cheating. I got 100%, and they still thought I cheated on it. For some reason, people look at me and just assumed I wasn't smart. If you think I can't do it, just watch me. I know I inherited that from my mom.

The one thing I can tell you about DTM was that there was no bullying at all. All the kids knew you just don't pick on the disabled kids. If there was even the slightest hint of it, teachers stepped in right away and put an end to it. With so many disabled kids throughout the school, they weren't shocked when I was in their class. I always felt welcomed. I think the biggest thing that helped me is my sense of humor. When I am nervous, or my anxiety shoots up, I always have had my sense of humor. Even if I had to get laughs by poking fun at myself, that's what I did.

DTM had these massive ramps instead of stairs that lead up to the top floor. There was a school aide that wheeled me to and from class. When in class, I was on my own. I remember being nervous if the other kids would even talk to me. They always did, and they still had a lot of questions. I always tried to answer them. The kids had seen other kids in wheelchairs in the school, but I was the only one in their class. I was just in math at first, and that was only an hour a day. Then I would go back to the disabled classes.

I remember feeling strange about how things were working. Around the disabled kids, they looked up to me because I got to go to regular classes. When I went to the regular classes, they welcomed me, but I was also an outsider who wasn't there much. I felt isolated, unsure where I fit, and I have times I feel the same way even now.

As I got older, it became evident to me that the world I lived in was different from just about everyone that I knew. My best friend at this time was Chuck. He sat next to me in the regular classes, and we became fast friends. The hard part came when the kids in my class all lived around the school while I did not. They would talk about everything they were doing hanging out after school. They had hung out together on weekends, and I was unable to do that. There were many times I wished I was like them, or I could hang out with them and do the things they were doing.

The summer before our 6th-grade year, Chuck wanted me to come over and spend the night. The only issue was talking my mom into it. The idea scared her because they weren't used to anyone in a wheelchair. I begged and begged, and finally, after talking to Chuck's dad several times, she finally said OK. I could tell she wasn't happy about it. The couple of days I spent at Chuck's house was the time of my life. He pushed me in my wheelchair all over the place. We went to other friends' houses, and we went to the local store. We played and had fun. We didn't do anything special when I look back on it. But that wasn't the point. I finally felt like a regular kid.

Just like other kids, I wanted to go to the school near where I lived. There was one problem we had. Fenton claimed they couldn't handle a student with disabilities. They had planned to still have me go to school in Flint. My mom didn't like this idea, so she started to argue with them. They gave up and said I could start going to Fenton in 7th grade. My mom went through the school. She made them put a ramp in. She also made sure the bathrooms were wheelchair accessible. She did the best she could to make sure the school would be ready. I was finally going to a school in the area where I lived. Thanks to my mom Fenton would be prepared for me. The real question was, I prepared for it.

Chapter 4

When I started Fenton, it was like I had rolled into another world. One that mentally, I was unprepared to handle. I walked with crutches at the time, but I couldn't walk for long distances. They got me a three-wheeled electric cart to ride around between classes. When I was at DTM, all the kids were used to seeing kids in wheelchairs. At Fenton, I was the only one, and I stuck out like a sore thumb. I was never stared at before, but now everywhere I went, that's all everyone did. It is hard enough starting a new school, not knowing anyone, but starting a new school as the only disabled kid was unbelievable. Add to it the fact that I was never really bullied in school before. I just was nowhere near ready for what I was facing. I was struggling from the word go, and it wasn't just the kids but the teachers and the principal too. It became clear to me that I wasn't wanted there. I think they thought that if they made it hard enough on me, I would want to go back to Flint.

Thankfully for me, though, I wasn't the only one starting in the school that day. I remember going to lunch. I was the first one in the lunchroom. I sat down and started to eat just trying to ignore all the kids staring. That's when Daron sat down across from me. He asked me my name, and we started talking. Daron had just moved to the area from Grand Rapids, and he didn't know anyone either. He needed a friend just as much as I did. We hit it off rather quickly. Then during the same lunch, Greg came and sat with us as well. He had moved to Fenton before the start of summer and didn't know many people. We became very close friends from then on.

Not long after my first marking period at Fenton, they made me take a series of tests. I think to try and prove that I couldn't do the work that was required so they could ship me back to Flint. They were a lot like the tests I took when I was younger at DTM. The tests took three days, and after them, we had a meeting with my mom. At the conference, they said I passed the tests with flying colors. The psychologist who gave them to me did say she was surprised by my intelligence.

The question became, why was I doing so poorly? I tried to explain to them all the bullying that had been going on. The superintendent and others did not want to believe anything that I had to say. The kids, especially the boys, were mean as they could get. They loved to kick my crutches out from under me as I was walking or grab my books and throw them. If I was in my three-wheeled cart, they tried to tip it over. They would stick their foot under the tire, and as I ran them over, they would complain to teachers.

I told them about what had been going on in my computer class. In that class, we all had assigned seats. My seat was in the first seat in the first row. I wasn't complaining about the desk I had. My issue was with who was around me. The boy behind me was one of my biggest bullies. The boy next to me was just as bad. Then there was the boy behind him who was as bad as the other two. They had me surrounded, and I did complain to the teacher who did nothing. He refused to even talk to the boys about what they were doing. They thought it was funny to spit on me all class long. You could see it on my desk and my books but still the teacher did nothing. Which, in turn, told the boys what they were doing was OK. Things just got worse from there.

I started getting what I now know is an anxiety attack going to that class every day. No one seemed to believe me in the meeting. They went and got the teacher. What the teacher had to say still has me dumbfounded to this day. He said that while some of the things may be going on in his class, it wasn't the fault of the boys. He said the mistake was mine. I was trying too hard to fit in. If I didn't work so hard to fit in, things would be easier on me.

I also learned early on that I couldn't go to the bathroom between classes. If I had to go, the safest time was during class when I would be the only one in there. The reason being is they loved to knock me down in the bathroom or accidentally pee on me. Or in some cases both. As I said, it just wasn't easy on me. The principal didn't like me, and he hated my three-wheeled cart. He told me not to drive it around because it wasn't safe for the other kids. When I complained to my mom, he said he would never tell me that. I knew I wouldn't be able to win with the principal and going to anyone for help would be pointless. I may have always had good grades up to this point. My grades in Fenton were terrible.

Not everything was all wrong, though. I had some great friends in Greg and Daron. We were spending the night at each other's houses and hanging out just about every chance we got. Usually, our base of operations seemed to be Greg's house. His house also had a bunch of neighbor kids up and down the street. There was always something going on. Greg's parents made everyone feel more than welcomed.

Not that I didn't feel welcomed at Daron's house because I did. It's just his dad was a preacher, and you had to watch what you said and did at his house. They didn't believe in dancing or going to the movies and that kind of thing. I am not saying there is anything wrong with that; it's just not for me. I think that is the one thing Greg did for both Daron and me. He forced us to come out of our shells. We had both grown up very sheltered and in controlled environments. We hadn't experienced much. Some may say Greg was a bad influence, but I wouldn't put it that way. He just showed us there was a lot more to life than we had seen so far. I couldn't have picked two better friends, especially on my first day when I was worried I might never make friends.

We did get in our fair share of trouble. We probably should have gotten in more, but we were lucky we didn't always get caught. As I think back at some of the things we did, all I can do is shake my head and laugh. Greg lived a few miles away, and at first, he would meet me at my house. Eventually, I would meet him halfway, or I would wheel all the way. That is something I never thought I would ever do before meeting Greg. He had a way of making me believe in myself and that I could do things that my mind said I couldn't. The three of us were all over town from one side to the other.

Usually, if we were at Greg's, we were playing outside with all the kids in the area. Sometimes we would play baseball in the back yard. I was always the umpire. When I called Greg out, and he didn't like the call, he would flip my chair backward and just kind of leave me that way for a few minutes. He didn't do it to be mean, though. Sometimes we played volleyball. They changed the rules so I could play. They allowed me to catch the ball and just throw it over the net. They always tried to make everything so that I could play as well. I don't remember a time where Greg and Daron didn't include me in whatever they wanted to do. We even went and played putt-putt golf together. It wasn't always easy getting my wheelchair in and out of places, but they were determined, and I always appreciated that.

I was also able to become close friends with a few girls as well. There were a few that would say mean things from time to time, but they were all friendly. For that reason, most of my friends were girls. In 7th grade, the two closest girls I made friends with were Theresa and Alexis. Alexis was in a few of my classes. She was a beautiful brunette with a peaceful, sweet demeanor about her. I have to admit I looked forward to classes we had together, and it had nothing to do with class. She was a real sweetheart. We never got as close as I would have liked. She at least brightened my day daily during a period I needed it.

Theresa, on the other hand. She was the kind of girl that will turn your world on its ear. She was a real wild child with a very free spirit. She was what some would say was a bad girl. Not that she did terrible things outside of maybe smoking. She just would say and do what she wanted. Theresa and I had the same group of friends, so it was natural that we would hang out. We talked on the phone almost every day for hours. It didn't take long for me to be head over heels for her. But I had another issue. Daron also liked her a lot and was talking to her. Not that I minded. Theresa had been clear with both of us. She wasn't interested in anything beyond friends with either of us. That, however, didn't stop us from trying.

When 8th grade started, I met Jeff. We had a lot in common we both loved video games and sports. Hanging out with Jeff was a little more complicated. He lived out in the country in the middle of nowhere. When we wanted to hang out, we had to rely on our parents. We were still a few years from driving. Hanging out with Jeff was different. He wasn't the outside type, so it seemed that everything we did was inside. It never really mattered to me.

I was doing OK at school, but I will admit I could always have done better than I did. I was way more focused on having fun than actually doing school work. I was still being bullied by the same kids all the time. My first hour was my most hated class. I didn't have any friends in the class. I was free game for the bullies. The teacher never really paid much attention. I know he saw and heard things he just chose not to do a damn thing about it. We had an end of the year project that was to be a group project. Each group was to have 3-4 kids per group. When it came time to choose groups, no one wanted me in their group.

The teacher did try and talk people into it, but no one would do it. I ended up doing a solo project when everyone else was in a group. I would like to say it didn't matter to me, but it did. I would like to say it didn't break me, but it did. I remember going home and crying that night. I felt I was as isolated and lonely as ever. And the kids were so cruel during that project. They would joke and laugh about it. I tried to ignore it but I couldn't. The teacher finally went off on the entire class, but by then it was too late. I wanted to skip that class every day. I still had to go, and I still had to finish the project. No kid should ever feel that way!

Chapter 5

At the start of high school, we had all gone to a football game and a dance after. I had danced with Theresa. I remember that she smelled of an intoxicating mixture of cigarette smoke and perfume. That combination now would make me want to throw up, but my hormones were all over the place. It had an odd effect on me. We all went outside and were hanging out with another one of my friends Darryl who was a junior. Theresa and Darryl were into each other, and I didn't take it well. I don't blame Theresa, though. She had been upfront and honest with me. It was my fault I didn't listen.

For days I felt like someone had punched me in the stomach. I just never let my mind even think about what would happen when Theresa started dating someone. And now seeing it with my own two eyes, it was a rough time. Greg and Daron did everything they could to try and cheer me up. My relationship with Theresa would never be the same again. After this, I kind of put a wall up and stayed my distance. We were still friends but not nearly as close as we were.

Theresa was the least of my worries. I had been to the doctor and found out I had to have major hip surgery. I hadn't had an operation in years. I thought they were behind me, and now this. The surgery was in January. With the operation hanging over my head, it's all that I had on my mind. The months passed, and before I knew it, I was in the hospital for my surgery. The surgery was rough. I would be in a body cast again. I had to be in the cast for four months. I wouldn't be able to move at all. There is no way to prepare yourself mentally for that. I was depressed and lonely. My friends did try and stop by when they could. They never stayed long, and I don't blame them. I really couldn't do much but watch TV or play video games, and that got boring.

I was at a low point in my life. All I wanted to do was go and hang out and do the things I used to do. I think it was that dream and doing all of that, which pushed me to get better. After I was out of my cast, I knew I had to keep going so I could hang out with my friends. As soon as I was able to get around a little bit better, my friends were there. I still remember my first day out. It was a fantastic spring day, and the air was warm and perfect. School was just about to let out, and summer was just around the corner. I spent that whole summer hanging out with my friends and preparing for my sophomore year.

One great thing that happened in my sophomore year was I had choir class. That is when I met Audra. I just remember her smile and eyes caught my attention right away. We sat close to each other and had plenty of time to talk. It wasn't long till we were good friends. Audra kind of fit into the spot in my life that Theresa had. I was talking to Audra all the time. I was starting to develop feelings that went beyond friendship. I did try and explore those. Audra was clear that she just wanted to be friends. I wasn't happy about it. I can't fault her for being honest with me. I loved the fact that I could count on her when I needed to talk. That didn't mean I wasn't jealous sometimes.

I found myself fighting jealousy quite often. I hated feeling that way; it just happened. I tried not to let it show too often, but sometimes it did. There is a scene in the movie The Fault in our Stars that explains my feelings perfectly. It's a small scene with no words, but I know the feelings in the scene. The scene is of Hazel sitting in the food court at the mall reading a book. She is having a drink by herself. She looks over and sees a girl about her age kissing her boyfriend. Hazel stares for a minute, then sighs and goes back to her book. I know what Hazel is thinking at that moment. She sees everything she has ever wanted, and yet Hazel fears she will never have. That movie and especially the book is the most accurate portrayal of kids with disabilities I have ever read or seen in a film. They did a fantastic job!

My dating life may have been a disaster but school was going much better. I was excited for my junior year. Half my day would be at high school and the rest at the skill center, which was a career style school in Flint for all the local area schools. I looked forward to getting away and taking classes in what I wanted to learn. Plus, to get away from all the bullying sounded like a great idea. I had fun in my skill center class, and with everyone all from different schools, it kind of took away all the usual clicks. The class was small, less than 20 kids in total. I knew one of the kids in the class and quickly made some other friends. The course was harder than I expected at first; it moved at a college pace.

While I was at the skill center, I met a girl in my class named Sara. Sara was timid at first. We started talking, and we became friends fairly quickly. With Sara, things went much slower for me than they had with Audra or Theresa. I think I was starting to grow up and mature. I had also put walls up to prevent myself from getting hurt. She knew she could count on me, and I would never hurt her. As Audra and I grew apart, I just really replaced her with Sara. We went out to dinner and a movie at least once a month. We even would go to family events together. If either of us needed a date for anything, we could always count on each other. I cared for her. I thought about being more than friends, but I never said anything to her about it. I believe in part because I was afraid I would ruin what we had.

Sara and I weren't in the same class in our senior year. We were at the skill center at the same time. We would see each other often, even if it was for a quick hi or a hug. I can honestly admit I did love Sara. I can't help, but wonder, would things be different had a spoken up and had I acknowledged it. I remember that toward the end of the school year, I wanted to go to prom. It was a dream of mine. It looked like fun to get all dressed up and go. But I knew I couldn't go stag. The kids already bullied me enough.

I knew had I even attempted to go stag; they would have made my life pure hell. I had asked Sara, but her prom was the same day, and she had already agreed to go with her boyfriend. I did ask Monica, who was in my skill center class. She said she would if it wasn't the same day as her, but it was. I just couldn't catch a break. I wish I could have thought of someone to ask at Fenton. I didn't think anyone would say yes. My mom tried to talk me into going anyway, but I just couldn't. I wish I would have been strong enough mentally just to say fuck it and go. I let too much of what the bullies said and did bother me. It honestly is my biggest regret in high school.

While in the Skill Center, I became friends with Clem. I had known Clem for years, but we never really hung out much. He also had a car which was huge. I no longer lived in town. I lived in Lake Fenton and really couldn't wheel anywhere. I think I spent every weekend at his house. Thankfully his mom was awesome and never seemed to mind. I was lucky not just that I had great friends, but their parents were just awesome to me. They all treated me like a member of the family.

Even Daron's parents, who were stricter than the others, couldn't have been kinder. I always expected at some point for some parents to ask why their son would want to hang out with me, but they never did. They always welcomed me, usually with a hug, and offered to stay for dinner. Because Clem's stepdad had a stroke, they even had a ramp on the front of their house. I joked with them a few times that they added that on just for me. As senior year winded down I needed to decide what my next step would be.

I had decided that the best college choice for me would be Ferris State University in Big Rapids, Michigan. They had a great business and computer department. It was also far enough away from home but not too far. My grandparents were only an hour away if I needed help. I started the application process and was accepted. Clem would also be going to Ferris. It made it helpful, knowing my best friend would be there with me. In May of 1990, I took my senior exams and had my last day in high school.

After all the bull shit and all the bullying, I was happy it was over. I think back at my time in high school whenever I see a kid who commits suicide after being bullied. People openly wonder how or why something like that can happen. I understand how desperate those kids were. You just get to a point where you need it to stop. You get to a point where you just want the pain to go away. I understand why they felt that was their only option. I wish they had stopped and reached out to someone. I know from personal experience that even if they had reached out, it doesn't mean anything would have changed.

On graduation night, the school had an all-night party for all the graduates called Project Graduation. I think it's a way for all the graduates to party and have a great time in a safe drug and alcohol-free environment. They had food, drinks, games, and dancing. Everyone was put on teams to play games. I was scared at first because of my experiences over the last six years.

I didn't think the kids would want me on their team or would even want me to play. They shocked me that night. All of the kids were encouraging me to play and also helping me at times. These weren't the same kids that I had known since my time at Fenton. They were the exact opposite. I even made out with a girl I had a crush on forever. Yes, it was a fantastic night. I couldn't help but wonder after the party why they couldn't have been that accepting in school. I do find it sad that my best day in high school just happened to be my last day.

Chapter 6

Getting ready for college was unlike anything I can explain. I was nervous but anxious and excited. I thought I was ready for the next step. My mom and I took a tour of the campus over the summer. I really couldn't wait to start the next phase of my life. I remember packing up my room, unsure of what I was going to be doing. I thought I would be able to get around by using my wheelchair. Because my wheelchair took up so much space, I was going to have my own room. I would be sharing a bathroom with someone who was also in a wheelchair. The bathroom itself was bigger than most dorm rooms with a complete roll-in shower. It was set up perfectly for me. The campus was huge, and everywhere had ramps and everything that I would need.

It wasn't long until it was a move-in day, and that was organized chaos. People from all over the state moving into the dorms and saying goodbye to their parents. I can't explain the overwhelming feeling of freedom I had after my mom left. I could go anywhere I wanted. I had no curfew for the first time. Honestly, for someone who grew up sheltered and isolated, it was too much of a good thing. Clem didn't live in my dorm, but he wasn't far away. On our first night there, we did what every red-blooded college kid recently set free would do. We went to the bar. We may have both just been 18, but finding someone over 21 willing to buy for us wasn't that difficult.

Once I was all moved in and settled, it was time to prepare for my first day of classes. I was a little nervous about getting to and from classes. I had wheeled long distances before, but I knew this would be different. My first class was a major disaster. My class was in the building that was the furthest out. It would take me a long time to get there. I wheeled out there. My class was on the 2nd floor. The problem was when I got there that the building was old and didn't have an elevator. How does that even happen? You would think that at least there would be some kind of warning. I was pissed! I couldn't believe I wheeled out there for nothing. I had to go to the councilor's office and fix my schedule.

Thankfully it didn't take long, and I was off again to my next class. I had a harder time wheeling around the campus than I expected. I was enjoying my new found freedom. It was also a lot to deal with at once. My procrastination issue was still going strong. I learned a valuable lesson. Once you get behind in college, it is almost impossible to catch back up. If you focus all your efforts on catching up in one class, then you're behind in two. Not to mention, I had a very active social life. For the first time, it seemed that just about everyone I met wanted to hang out and party. I am not going to lie. I lived it up. The problem is you can't have good grades in college and an overactive social life. I was burning the candle at both ends, and I paid the price.

With winter rapidly approaching, I knew getting around would be a big problem. I started asking the school what options I had. They said that if I had someone that could wheel me around, they would set it up so that we would be able to schedule our classes first. Usually, scheduling went by seniority so that first-year students would schedule last. Sometimes you had to fight to get a class you wanted. But this would make it much more manageable.

I talked to Clem, and he was OK with it, so we set that up. I also learned that because I was disabled, I could get clearance to have a car on campus. I didn't have a car at the time, but Clem did. Now we had a car on campus as well. Turns out, being in a wheelchair wasn't all bad. Even if I wasn't hanging out with Clem, I was hanging out with my other friends in my dorm. I didn't have a roommate, so if anyone was having issues with theirs, they came to my room. I don't remember sleeping much. I was instead more focused on having fun, and that's what I did.

College isn't just about having fun. I knew I needed to focus more on school. In my second term, I came to learn one valuable piece of information. I hated computer programming. I thought I would love it because I loved computers. I had never actually tried programming. When I started programming, I found it made me miserable. First of all, I type slowly, which for a computer programmer is a bad thing. Then a computer programmer has to love sitting in the lab for hours just programming. They don't talk or move;

they just program. I am a talker, and I love to talk to anyone. I will even talk to myself. I quickly found out that talking isn't allowed in the computer lab.

I started to get depressed because I didn't know what to do. The more depressed I got, the more I drank. Admittedly I was losing myself. I didn't want to admit I needed help. I was so stupid, and I just kept on the same path. I passed my classes but barely. I should have checked into changing my major, but I didn't do that. I stayed on the computer programming track even though I hated it. My next term was even worse.

The more advanced the classes got, the more miserable I was. My last straw for computer programming was when I was working on a project, and it wouldn't work. It took two computer lab assistants and me almost three hours to find a space that was in the wrong spot. I had something that had two spaces in between, and there was only supposed to be one. At that moment, I looked at myself in the mirror, and I knew this was not the life for me. I was going to have to make a change.

Clem and I realized it was expensive to have a social life in college. We decided to start our business selling sports memorabilia. It involved two of my favorite things. I loved talking to people, and I loved sports. It was an excellent combination for me. We started small and worked our way up. I learned people would buy and deal with people they trust. If you're friendly and trustworthy, people will come back. We had a business license and everything. We managed to do several shows in different states and even a couple in Canada.

The business was doing great, so we decided to go on a trip for spring break. We were on our way to lunch, and there was this travel company offering cheap cruises to the Bahamas. We put a deposit on the trip. We would get a one day cruise to the Bahamas. Then three days on the island and cruise back. There were a few bonuses to the trip to the Bahamas. First off, they don't have a drinking age. We would be able to drink legally. The Bahamas also had some excellent casinos so we would be able to gamble as well. Clem wanted to spend a few extra days in Florida. We added a day before and a day after the cruise.

I love to fly, but the hard part when you are disabled is getting on and off the plane. There is no easy way to do it. Planes just aren't designed for disabled people. Thankfully I had Clem with me. He had been used to helping me get around for years. He just grabbed me and pulled me onto the plane and threw me into a seat. They brought my chair up as far as they could, and he drug me off. We got our bags from the baggage claim, and the hotel had a van from the airport. The van wasn't wheelchair accessible. So getting in it was a struggle, but we managed to make it work.

We had a free day then we would be traveling to the Bahamas the following morning. There wasn't much to do around the hotel, and Clem wanted to go to the beach. The problem was the beach was 5 miles away. We tried only to spend money when we had to. Clem decided he was going to walk and push my wheelchair the entire way. We spent the day at the beach. That is real friendship right there, no doubt about it!

The next morning we had to get up early to catch a bus to the ship. We got to the boat and went through customs. We would just be on the ship for a few hours. We decided to roam the ship and check it out. The casino and bar wouldn't be open until we were in international waters. I quickly realized was that cruise ships are not wheelchair accessible. We tried to take the elevator. It was so small. Clem had to lift the back of the chair, so I was almost standing straight up. Then turn it to get us both in.

Soon we were in international waters, and we could drink and gamble. All I did was play the slots. We made it into port, and it was time to leave the ship. We ended up taking a ferry to the hotel, which took a few people helping to get the chair on. The next day we had booked a tour through the botanical gardens. We also had a tour of the town and shopping areas. I am glad we went; it was stunning. You got to see many styles of plants they didn't have in America.

We went to the shopping district and ended up picking up a bottle of Bacardi 151. Before we left the Bahamas, we acknowledged we had a problem. We still had half of the bottle of 151 left. We weren't going to let that go to waste. We went to the store and found a bottle of ginger ale that was close in color. Then we dumped it out and rinsed the bottle.

We poured the 151 into the ginger ale bottle. They took our luggage from us and had all the dogs sniff it. I am assuming looking for drugs. We were a bit worried because we saw them tell some people to open up their luggage. Had we done that, we would have in big trouble. The custom agents told us to grab our bags and go to an agent. As soon as we got to the agent, they looked at us asked us a couple of questions and waved us on. We walked calmly to the bus and went back to our hotel. Thankfully when we got back to the hotel, the bottle didn't break in transit.

When I went back to Ferris for my sophomore year, I was miserable. My mom had warned me if I didn't start doing better, she was going to make me move back home. I was already in that situation because I was under academic probation. The problem was I had dug myself into a hole already. I did work very hard in the term. I just couldn't figure out what I wanted to study. I was lost, but I was fighting.

I wasn't partying as much, but I couldn't stop drinking. I did try and cut back, but when the pressure got to me, I would drink. Then I would just get more depressed. It was a vicious cycle! I did a little better this term, but my grades weren't good enough. I had to move back home. I am still ashamed of how all this worked out. So many times, I think back to things I should have and could have done differently.

Chapter 7

After coming home from college, I was depressed and lost. I just didn't know what to do. My mom wanted to send me to rehab. But I refused and just quit cold turkey. It wasn't easy to do, but it was something I had to do. There were times I wanted to give up, but that isn't in my nature. I battled and overcame it. I registered for classes at Mott Community College in Flint. It was like starting over, but I was starting over much smarter and wiser. I planned to take a bunch of different classes and see what happens, and that's what I did.

I wasn't nervous about starting classes at Mott. I had already taken college classes, so I knew I could do the work. I was also sober by this point. I was looking forward to seeing what kind of grades I could get. I was nervous about the fact that I didn't know anyone. I have severe social anxiety when I am around people I don't know. On my first day after my first class, I decided to go down to the cafeteria and get some lunch. Much to my surprise, when I entered the cafeteria, there was another guy in a wheelchair. He was sitting at a table surrounded by several people. He looked familiar, but I wasn't sure what his name was. He saw me and instantly invited me to join them. Come to find out we had gone to DTM together many years ago. His name was Mike, and he quickly introduced me to everyone at the table.

I spent most of my free time playing cards with Mike and a small group of friends. My first crush of the group was Emilie. I have a thing for short girls, and she was short and a real sweetheart with a super bubbly personality. I was attracted to her as soon as I met her, and she knew it. We even went out a few times. The problem was she was still in love with her ex-boyfriend and wasn't looking for anything serious.

We also went out on a lot of group dates. We went bowling a few times. We had a party at Emilie's house. I have to admit I enjoyed hanging out with the group. It was nice to feel accepted. I would even go to Mott on the days I didn't have a class to hang out. No matter how rough of a day I had, I always felt better around them. They could make me smile and laugh, no matter what was going on. The group helped me overcome my problems with alcohol. I was no longer looking to drown my sorrows in a bottle.

Another member of the group was Carley. My first impression of Carley was that she was the biggest bitch I had ever met. I didn't like her at all. Although I have always found bitchy to be an attractive quality. Part of the problems I had with Carley was I couldn't figure out what her story was. When I first met her, I thought she was dating a guy named Jim. She would hang on him at school. I also knew they would hang out away from school. But she would also talk about her boyfriend named Ronald. It was somewhat confusing to me.

After talking with her, I got more of the story. Her relationship with Ronald was on the rocks, and all he was interested in was sex. She was just friends with Jim and not interested in more from him. She seemed almost to be as lost as I was. Just someone is searching for happiness and not sure what to do. At this point, my feelings for Emilie had died down a bit.

Things all started changing at one of our group bowling dates. We were all there and having a great time. I noticed that Carley was hanging around me more than usual. Not that I was complaining. The more we talked, the more we realized we had in common. Carley did tell me she had a son, and he was two. His name was Noah. I think she was testing me to see my reaction. I didn't have an issue with the fact that she had a son. After all, I have always loved kids, and they seemed to love me as well.

We talked a lot about our home lives and how miserable we were. She wasn't happy, and she wanted to move out desperately. One thing I had been thinking about was my aunt worked as the manager for a new apartment complex. She had a handicapped accessible unit that would be open soon if I wanted it. The only issue was I couldn't afford the rent on my own. I would need a roommate to help me cover the costs. I had asked a few friends, but to this point, no one was willing to do it. The ones that were I didn't think were that reliable. I didn't mention it to Carley, but the idea was already in my head.

After the group bowling date, Carley and I started spending more and more time together. I had met her mom several times because she worked at the college. Meeting her dad was a memorable experience. When he walked through the door, the whole mood of the house would instantly change. It would go from a happy go lucky to more of a doom and gloom situation. He just had an angry aura around him. Even Noah would change. One minute he would be a happy and laughing toddler, and then when Carley's dad came home, Noah would instantly turn to a crying fussy kid, which would immediately set her dad off. He would yell and make the situation worse.

That's another thing he never really talked to anyone. All he seemed to do is yell. He ran the house with fear. Later Carley would tell me stories of many times he had gotten physical with her. He loved to threaten Noah if he didn't stop crying. This made me angry. My real dad had abused me. I felt the need to protect them and take care of them.

That's when I started mentioning to Carley about moving into the apartment with me. I felt like it would work out well. I needed a roommate, and she needed a way out of her house. Noah needed a positive father figure. I knew I could do that. I had always wanted kids, and to be honest, it didn't matter to me that he wasn't mine by blood. All I knew is there was a child who didn't have a dad much like I didn't when I was growing up. I knew that feeling, and it sucked. This was my chance to be the dad I never had. I was starting to get excited about the future. Carley seemed to like the idea of moving in with me. She made it clear she just wanted to be friends.

My friends at Mott were giving me a lot of grief about my relationship with Carley. I guess the role I was now playing was a frequent one. She could draw guys in and yet still keep them at a certain distance. She would play with their emotions until they got mad and backed away. They told me I was the 4th or 5th guy to go through this.

Mike had been through the same thing with her a few months before I joined the group. He wanted to make sure I was careful. While I appreciated their concern, all the jokes and name-calling were annoying. I just wanted people to be happy for me. I knew we were moving way to fast. We had only been hanging out for a couple of months, yet we were talking about moving in together. Not to mention the fact that she still dating Ronald

Carley and I were growing closer by the day. We hadn't had sex, yet we had been fooling around. I was over her house; we were sitting on her bed, cuddling and watching a movie. Ronald had gotten out of work early decided to stop by. I happened to look up to see him standing in her doorway with a very shocked look on his face. He stormed out, and Carley chased after him. She left for several minutes. When Carley came back, she said Ronald wasn't happy. Carley denied that she was cheating on him. She was trying to convince him that we were just friends. With the position we were in when Ronald walked in, I doubt he was going to buy that. I was a bit upset over the fact that Carley was still saying we were just friends.

My mom wasn't thrilled with the idea of Carley and me moving in together. I had been honest with my mom about the situation. She just didn't want me to get hurt. She also knew that I wanted to move out on my own. She just wanted to make sure I knew what I was doing. She wanted to make sure that I was ready for all the responsibility with Noah.

I thought I was ready for everything. Our apartment was available in early June. We didn't have a lot of money between the two of us. My mom paid our security deposit to help us along. I appreciated the fact that she was willing to help us out. Even though she didn't approve, she wanted me to be happy, and she was ready to help me if I needed it.

We moved in during the second week of June with the help of our families. We didn't have much furniture, but we had enough for now. My family bought us some groceries to get us started, and we were all set. I still remember the first night in the apartment. It was exhilarating to be in our place and together. It was a two-bedroom apartment with two bathrooms. I had my bedroom with a separate bathroom complete with everything all wheelchair accessible. Then the 2nd bedroom had an attached bathroom. We set the 2nd bedroom up as Noah's, and we moved into the first bedroom. By now, we had been sleeping together for about a month. Carley was still trying to claim we were just friends again, but it didn't seem like that to me. She claimed she was still dating Ronald.

We had lived there for about a week, and things were going great. Until Carley told me that Ronald was coming over, he would be spending the night. I was pissed off. We had our first fight, and it was a long time coming. Carley said she had made it clear to me we were just friends. And while she had told me that she had also been sleeping with me. We were acting as a family, and you can't have it both ways. I was angry, and I didn't hide it. I wanted Ronald to know I didn't want him in my house.

I remember Noah kept coming into my room. He wasn't used to me not playing with him and spending time with him. When they went to bed, I almost lost my mind. I wanted to beat the shit out of Ronald. I was also angry at Carley. I have no clue how you can say you care about someone but do something like this. Noah cried and threw a fit all night. I could hear him, and for once, I wanted him to cry. I could also hear Carley and Ronald get in several fights over the situation. Thankfully they broke up a few weeks later. Although it was not the last time, Carley would remind me that we were just friends.

One time I remember was we went to a friend's wedding. We were both invited, but I barely knew this couple. I was Carley's date at the start of the wedding. By the time we got to the reception, she had reminded me that we were just friends. I went and got a drink when she said that. I knew damn well I was in for a long night. I only knew two people at this wedding. That was friends of ours, Kirk and Amy. Carley had seen another friend was there. His name was Rob. What was supposed to be a happy occasion to celebrate a wedding was turning into a miserable evening for me. Carley started out ignoring me and hanging on Rob and then dancing with him. They even went outside so he could smoke.

Kirk and Amy knew I was upset and did everything they could to calm me down. Amy went outside and tried to talk to Carley about what she was doing. People from the wedding who I didn't know were even making comments to Carley. They wondered why her boyfriend was inside, and she was hanging on Rob. She told them I was just a friend. She could have gone to this wedding without me. I may not have liked the idea, but at least I wouldn't have to watch her hang all over this guy.

There was not nearly enough alcohol in the world that night to calm me down. It took everything I had not to cause a scene at the wedding. We did get in a huge fight later because, to me, it was total bull shit. When we were at home, she was very caring. She told me she loved me. But at times when we were out in public, she would introduce me at times as her boyfriend and at other times as her friend. I never really felt comfortable. What I meant to her seemed to change depending on where we were and who was there.

After a while, Carley didn't say were just friends to anyone anymore. We were getting closer. For once, I was happy. I was doing well in college and getting close to graduating, as was Carley. Carley had gotten a job working at Blockbuster. Noah was also doing well. He seemed to be blossoming in a stable home environment. It was nice to be able to count on Carley the way I should have been able to from the start. I loved being a daddy to Noah. I will never forget the first time he called me daddy. My heart almost melted right there on the spot.

When I got approved for financial aid at Mott, I also got approved for federal work-study. That allowed me to get an on-campus job. I was excited about this because it would also give me valuable work experience that I needed. I went to the financial aid office and handed in my paperwork. I asked them about the work-study job. They told me I would have to talk to the job placement office. The placement office told me I had to go through a seminar explaining the program. Then I would meet with the work-study coordinator.

The work-study coordinator's name was Laura. I liked her right away. I explained how I had wanted a job and how hard it was. She was impressed with all the computer skills I had. She had a couple of posts that may fit me. She said one job was in the job placement office. They were looking for students to work 20 hours a week. I would have to interview with the department director. Her name was Karen, and she couldn't meet with me till the next day.

I arrived early for my interview with Karen. I know you are supposed to be early, but I was even earlier than that. It gave me a chance to look around the office. I played around on a few of their computer programs to see how they worked. Soon it was time for my interview. I was struck by how different

Karen was to Laura. While Laura was slightly sweet and calm and spoke softly, Karen was the exact opposite.

Karen wasn't mean just one of those women you want to stay on her good side. I liked her, and I thought the interview went well. After I got home, I got a call from Laura that I had gotten the job. I was so excited I kept thanking her. I wasn't as much enthusiastic about the money as I was the work experience that was far more valuable.

I loved the job from the start. The office had several departments. Each had a separate manager, but everyone was in the same office. They had on-campus jobs, off-campus jobs, internships, and the educational and research side. If an employer wanted to post a job, we would fax them the forms to fill out. For anyone on work-study, we would sign them up to meet with Laura and make sure their paperwork was in order.

We could only work a max of 20 hours a week on the program, and I worked every hour I could. I would even go in if I had time to kill between classes. I got yelled at for working off the clock on several occasions. I just loved working, so that's what I did. Karen told me it was a violation of the program, and they could get in trouble. I would apologize then end up doing it anyway. I was doing it on my own free will, so it shouldn't be a problem. I was thrilled, and Laura seemed to love my work, as well. She had me write up training manuals for the office. When they hired new staff each term, I was the one who trained them.

My life seemed to be falling into place finally. I had a job I loved even if I wasn't making much money while doing it. School was going well. I was getting A's in all of my classes. My home life was terrific, as well. Noah was growing daily and blossoming into a happy child. He was so different than when I first met him. I couldn't even believe he was the same kid. I was amazed at how a simple change of environment had affected him. Carley and I were even talking about taking the next step in our relationship.

Chapter 8

After being together for almost two years, Carley and I started talking about getting married. I was very open to the idea. We hadn't had any issues in over a year. Carley said she would like to have another child as well. She wanted the kids to be close in age, and Noah was four now. I loved the idea of having a child of my own. Don't get me wrong. I considered Noah mine. I loved him very much, but I knew having a blood-related child would be different.

I thought it would take Carley longer to get pregnant than it did. I came home from work a few months later, and there was a pregnancy test on the table. I really couldn't have been happier. I couldn't believe it at first. It was near my birthday and a few weeks away from Christmas. I couldn't imagine a better present. I couldn't wait to tell the rest of the family. I had never been so happy in my life. My life was finally going the way that I had always wanted. I couldn't imagine life being much better than this. Life wasn't perfect but it was close.

I will be the first to admit having another child probably wasn't the best idea we ever had. While we were getting by, we didn't have a lot of money. With a baby on the way, things were going to get very tight. Especially when the baby was born because Carley would have to take time off of work, we needed all the money we were making right now. Carley said she could get more hours at Blockbuster, and I decided to look for a better part-time job.

I got called about one of my resumes I had sent out through the placement office. The job was 2nd shift at a bank as a proof encoder. The job was to process checks after the bank closed and put the dollar amount on the bottom in magnetic ink. You sat at a giant machine with a number pad on it. We would read the amount on the check and type in the amount and run the check through the machine. It would add the amount on the bottom in magnetic ink. We would add up the amount of checks and put the account number and the amount in magnetic ink on the deposit slip.

I had several issues with this job from the start. First off we couldn't talk while working. If you got caught talking, the bank would yell at you and even write you up. The next issue was the office itself was not wheelchair friendly. All the banks sent the checks for processing in huge bags. As the bags came in, they were emptied and just thrown around. They had huge electrical cords for the machines run all over. When I went to get checks to process, I had to wheel over all the cords and the bags. I asked several times if people could just bring them to me, but they said no.

They paid me by the hour, but our hourly rate depended on how many checks we processed when I got stuck going to get checks, which would dramatically affect my hourly rate. Carley had a cousin Jane that worked in the same office. She tried several times to help me. They made it clear no one was to help me. The job also had a rate objective that I had to reach each month, or they would write me up. Because I was new, the goals started very small and then ramped up.

The last issue was the parking situation. We worked late at night, and the building was in downtown Flint. The bank wanted us to park in the attached parking garage. I couldn't park there because it was an old building and it didn't have any ramps for wheelchairs. Every entrance off of the parking garage had stairs. I was shocked and had never seen anything like it. I pointed out the issue the bank managers were not even aware of the situation. They had just assumed there was an acceptable entrance. That meant I had to park across the street in a parking lot. Once after a massive snowstorm, I got my wheelchair stuck trying to cross the road in snow and almost got hit by a car.

This was far from my dream job. I was starting to realize that I may be in over my head. I did try and talk to my manager Angela to explain the issues. I had some research on the laws for the employment of disabled people. I knew that they had to try and make some concessions as far as trying to make it easier to get the checks. I even demonstrated how hard it was to get around the office. I knew from her tone I was screwed. As the weeks went on, I did the best I could. I even saw them yell at people who would grab extra work and drop it off to me. My numbers were OK but not great. They were behind the other new employees.

I was not at our goal after the first month. My boss Angela called me into the office and told me I had to work harder. I pointed out the issues, and she said they wouldn't do anything about them. Angela said it was my issue, and I had to figure it out. I tried to point out what the laws said, but she wasn't having any of that. I was getting beyond frustrated.

The 2nd month didn't go much better for me. I had done better than the first month, but I was still behind. I had another meeting with Angela. She pointed out that I was behind the objective still. She made it clear that I had to be at goal for the final month, or they would fire me. I asked if it would have been possible to transfer to another position within the bank. She said that she would look into it. By the tone of her voice, I doubted seriously she would do it.

The writing was on the wall, and I needed to try and do something. I decided to go in the morning and talk to the job placement office. Laura suggested that I speak to the off-campus job coordinator. I went and spoke to her and spilled the entire story. Her name was Bonnie. Bonnie wasn't thrilled with how the bank was treating me. She told me that the hotel downtown had new ownership. They were hosting a job fair.

I met with the human resource director of the hotel. Her name was Michelle, and we got along really well. She explained that her company had just bought the hotel. They had plans to renovate and hire all new staff. They needed a lot of people, especially in the front desk and reservations area. The job sounded right up my alley. She was looking for full-time employees, especially if I was willing to work weekends. I told her I would work where ever and whenever they wanted me to.

Michelle called me and asked if I could come in for another interview with the front desk manager. I made arrangements to meet with Jeffrey. They said Jeffrey was in a meeting and was running behind when I arrived. I had already been waiting for a half-hour when I started to get a bit nervous. I had to get to work at the bank. I was beginning to think I was going to be late. I doubted the bank would give a shit if I showed up at all. I knew they would fire me soon.

I called the bank and told them I was at a doctor's appointment, and it was running late. Just as I was talking to them, Jeffrey walked in. Here I was calling in late to my current job while at an interview for my new job. I knew this was not a good look for me. Jeffrey apologized for keeping me waiting. I made a joke of wishing I had made a better first impression. He told me not to worry about it. He said he understood, and it was his fault for making me wait. The interview with Jeffrey went well. We ended up talking about his thoughts on my role and his plans for the future of the hotel. I was excited about the possible opportunity.

After the interview, I headed to the bank. I ended up being about 20 minutes late. They weren't happy, and I didn't give a damn. A week later, I had just gotten to work; they told me I had to go down to human resources. I went down to the office and waited for human resources to talk to me. The longer I waited the madder I got. Her name was Paula. She started off telling me that I was the only one in the office below target. She said they wanted me to take a voluntary layoff. They would look for another job for me within the bank. Paula actually wouldn't guarantee that they would ever find a job for me.

I knew had I taken the voluntary layoff. I wouldn't have been able to get unemployment. I said no to the voluntary lay off. I went through all the issues I had getting around the office. I explained how that shouldn't have counted against me. I told Paula how many times I had talked to Angela and how she denied any assistance. I went so far as to say to her what the law says about my situation. She was speechless at this point. She said that if I didn't take the voluntary layoff, they would fire me. I told her to fire me!

I was worried about the future. I just really hoped the hotel would call soon. I just sat down to eat dinner, and the phone rang. It was Michelle from the hotel. Michelle said she was calling to offer me the job. They wanted me to start Monday afternoon. I hung up the phone and laughed because it really couldn't have worked out better. I was only unemployed for about an hour.

I was supposed to start at the hotel on Monday, but they called me on Friday. They asked if I would start that afternoon and work for the weekend. They wanted me to come in and talk to Jeffrey so I would understand the role they had for me. I had a great feeling about my possible future at the hotel. I arrived, and Jeffrey was waiting for me. He showed me around and introduced me to everyone. I would be mainly 2nd shift. My main title would be a phone operator. I would primarily handle calls coming into the hotel. I would also handle any guest calls and send up housekeeping or maintenance. Jeffrey also wanted me to do a bit more than that. He wanted me to learn the reservation system and start doing them when the reservations manager wasn't there. I started right then and worked all that day.

It didn't take me long to learn the phone and their computer system. I worked the entire weekend. I met the reservations manager Catherine. My meeting with her did not go according to plan. She made it clear she didn't want me making any reservations. She wouldn't give me access to the reservations system. She wasn't about to teach me anything. She treated me like an invading enemy. I left her office and went to Jeffrey's office. He asked me how it went, and I laughed and told him what had happened. He told me I was doing a great job and just to keep up the great work. I needed to hear that.

When I had first started at the hotel, the general manager was named Will. He kind of let the front desk staff do their own thing, and he left us alone. After I had been there for a few months, the new owners brought in someone new as the GM. His name was Percy and he came from another property in California. Because he lived in California, he lived in the hotel while he was GM. The best way I can describe him is to imagine Donald Trump with a Greek accent.

I had never met someone so arrogant and narcissistic in my life. Percy acted like he could treat anyone how he wanted. He would say anything to anyone, and they couldn't do a damn thing about it. I saw Percy chase down guests to yell at them for smoking in the lobby while he was smoking in the lobby. God help them if they dared point out he was smoking too. He would get in their face and start screaming. Not long after Percy got there, Jeffrey quit. Percy decided to promote Catherine and then move me to the reservations manager. He also wanted me to learn the front desk.

When I got promoted to the reservations manager, they put me on salary. This was good and bad at the same time. The good part was I would be making more money. The bad part was I would be working a minimum of 50 hours a week. What I didn't know at the time, but I learned quickly was the 50 hours a week would be a pipe dream. I would end up working way more than that. The way it worked out, Catherine and I were killing ourselves. They had fired or laid off a lot of the staff. They left only six people to cover the front desk 24 hours a day, seven days a week.

One problem I had with the reservations job was upper management wanted everything done their way. Catherine had worked there for 20 years and was still doing the job the same way. She typed up all her reports on a manual typewriter. I tried it her way, but it was crazy and very time-consuming. I am from the computer age with a computer programing background. I wanted to modernize the whole thing, and they didn't. I couldn't see the point of manually typing up a forecast report every week.

They fought me on it for months till I finally just did it my way. I wrote up all-new programs. I was able to give updated numbers at the drop of a hat. I had to save time where I could. I was doing two jobs and only getting paid for one. Catherine and I were working most of the hours. She worked all morning shifts, and I worked the afternoon and evening shifts. We had no choice but to work every day. We both had worked 80 days straight. We were exhausted! We then tried every two weeks; one of us would work a double and give the other a day off. The hard part of working at a hotel, especially as management, is it never closes.

Chapter 9

Not long after the hotel promoted me, my daughter Lys was born. I remember almost every little detail of the whole day. It was the happiest day of my entire life. I can't even really describe the feeling. I remember the first time I held her. When she opened her eyes and looked at me, I swear my heart smiled. She stole my heart the first seconds she was alive. I looked into her eyes, and I said I would never leave her, and I would always be there for her. I was bound and determined to be the best dad I could be. I promised to be the dad to her that I didn't have. When Lys was born, I knew I had to straighten up and do right by her. Not that I hadn't already done that for Noah, but it was different now. I was just glad she was born happy and healthy. That was by far the most important thing.

After Lys was born, not much changed. For the most part, she was a great baby. On the rough nights, it made work the next day a little long. I took a week of vacation right after Lys was born, and Carley stayed off work for a month. We were also planning our wedding. The wedding was still a year away. We had talked many times about just going to the courthouse and just getting married and calling it good. Both of our families wanted a bigger wedding with a reception. They all promised to pitch in where they could. Both sides offered to pay for specific parts, and Carley's aunt promised to do our pictures for free. Carley's uncle owned a bakery, so we got a cake for cost. We also got a discount on catering and the hall. Things were falling into place.

I was now working a lot of hours at the hotel. Carley also got a promotion at Blockbuster. Neither of us liked the added hours, but we needed the money. It didn't give us much time for each other, but we were parents. As far as I was concerned, it was more about the kids than it was about us

A couple of weeks before Christmas, I was shocked to get called in and told the hotel had to lay me off. They made it clear that my layoff was just temporary. My time off didn't last long, however. A few days after Christmas, I got a call, and I was back on the schedule. I wasn't a manager anymore. They wanted me part-time and hourly. I said OK because it was better than nothing and went back to work.

Percy came down and welcomed me back with a handshake. He said he was the one who demanded they bring me back. I thanked him and told him that I appreciated it. I worked a week on hourly pay. Then they put me back on salary with the convention coming in. Percy came to me a few times, telling me he was going to fire Catherine and promote me. He asked if I could do it. I said yes, I could. I was already working the hours, so I doubted anything would change. Catherine must have known what was coming. She quit before the convention even started. I couldn't blame her. She was taking a lot of heat for things that weren't her fault. Percy never took the blame for anything. It was always someone else's fault.

Taking over was a more significant change than I expected. I was Percy's target for abuse now. When I say abuse, which is what it was. He said things to me; you should never say to a disabled person even if you were joking. His favorite saying was, "If you can't move faster than that, then you need to get up and walk!" He loved to threaten to push me over, and he was not joking. He would even do it in front of guests. I had guests come to my defense, and he would then go off on them. He loved pointing out he was the GM. He loved knowing he had power. He knew I had to provide for my family. He used that against me. My hours went up even more now. To make matters worse, the hotel forced me to work alone, even when we were busy. I would work 12 hours or more with no breaks for the bathroom or the ability to eat. I was killing myself, and I knew it. I just didn't know what to do.

After that, my relationship with Percy got worse. He would go out of his way to make my life a living hell. He would call me at the front desk several times a day and mock me for not moving fast enough. He would call me retarded or worse. He would stand off to the side, and if he thought I was getting behind, he would start yelling. He acted as if the guests weren't even there. The sad part was the owners knew how he was. Several times the owners called me personally and admitted they knew he was abusive. They would say I was doing a great job, especially in an impossible situation. I will never understand why they let him get away with it. I heard him call African American employees monkeys as many times, and he called me retarded. Looking back at it now, I feel so stupid for putting up with all of it. I worried that finding another job would be impossible.

My life was a chaotic mess. I was working far too many hours in a hostile environment. I was trying to be a dad and plan a wedding. The wedding was going to be beyond our means. We were cashing in every favor we could to pull it off. We paid all the deposits and had made some other small payments to try and spread out the costs as much as possible. We had been planning and paying for almost a year.

Carley's parents kept saying their part of the money would be given to us soon. Two weeks before we had to have everything paid, they told us they couldn't give us any of the money. We were going to be screwed. If we canceled the wedding, we would lose all the deposits we had already paid. We had sent out the invitations already. This was going to be a mess. We did about the only thing we could think of doing. We took out a loan from the bank. We didn't want to do it, but it seemed like the most logical thing to do.

Carley did not want me in my wheelchair for the ceremony. She insisted that I be standing using my crutches during the ceremony. We would have my wheelchair standing by if I needed it. All I could think of the whole time was don't fall over. I was able to stay on my feet, and we were married. I will admit something, though. You would think my thoughts would have been about how happy I was. Or how excited I was for the future, but it wasn't.

My first thought was, "I wonder how long this will last." The honest and straightforward answer is I admit I settled. I settled for someone that would be with me. I knew neither of us was honestly happy. I did love Carley, and I did think that she loved me. Deep down, I knew it wouldn't last. Her history of behavior had told me that. We hadn't had issues in years. I knew she would act as she did in the past. My family knew this too, and my mom begged me not to marry her. I was sure if I loved her enough, she wouldn't cheat on me. I think on some levels; I lied to myself.

The reception is where things went a bit haywire. I guess when you mix people with alcohol sometimes that happens. We made sure we had an open bar. Things started fine, and we had great food and an excellent DJ. Before I knew it was already time to cut the cake. We had our first dance, and I danced with my mom and everyone was having a great time. Then all hell started to break loose.

Noah started acting up a bit. Instead of letting Carley or I take care of him, Carley's dad tried to take charge. He ended up spanking Noah hard in front of everyone which started people arguing. We tried to calm the situation, but it didn't work, and Carley ended up in tears. I know her family didn't like me, and my family wasn't exactly thrilled with Carley. I wish they could have put all that aside and just let us have our day. But I guess that was just too much to ask.

Once the wedding was over, I hoped that life would calm down. Percy, however, had different ideas. After my wedding, he was furious at me. He had wanted me to have my wedding at the hotel. I refused because he wouldn't give me a discount. He then stepped up his attacks on me. One day Percy came up to me and said my vehicle was a piece of shit. He didn't like it parked in front of the hotel. I told him I would happily get another vehicle if he would like to pay me more. He told me I couldn't park in front of the hotel anymore. I pointed out that is where the handicapped spaces were, and he couldn't tell me I couldn't park there.

The other parking for the hotel was in an attached parking garage. To get my wheelchair from the parking garage to the hotel would take 30 minutes. I was going to park where it was easier. One time Percy got mad at me about parking out front. He called a tow truck to tow me. I went out front when the tow truck got there. I warned the driver if he towed a legally parked handicapped vehicle, he would be in a world of hurt. He asked Percy why he wanted it towed. Percy told the guy the truth, and he refused to do it. That pissed Percy off. He tried to get others to tow me, but no one would. He then tried to make it company policy that employees couldn't park out front. I parked out front anyway.

Percy was a paranoid person, as well. He was sure the employees were out to rob the hotel blind. So instead of hotel security in place for the quests safety, he put them in the basement to keep an eye on the employees. One night when the hotel was slow, someone robbed me. Security saw the whole thing on video but couldn't get up to me in time. I just let them take the money seeing it was only a few hundred dollars. Percy didn't see it that way, though. He docked my check the amount that was stolen and wrote me up.

I was tired of getting screamed at all the time. Then the hotel hired a couple of new people. I knew something was up. I just didn't know what. We had a convention coming in, and I had a lot of work to do. One day before the convention, I was working late, making sure everything was ready when the night shift guy came in. He said he needed to talk to me, but he had to wait until everyone else was gone. He told me he spoke to the new guy that had been hanging around the reservations office. The new guy said the hotel hired him to be a new manager. The plan was to have me train him, and then they were going to fire me. This was like a kick to the gut.

I didn't sleep well that night because I had a lot to think over. I didn't have to work until 4 PM the next day. I had time to figure it out. I was looking forward to watching the Michigan vs. Penn St Football game before going into work. I knew what time I needed to start getting ready. I decided that if Michigan were leading at halftime, that would mean I should quit. If Penn St was winning, then that meant I should go into work. Michigan destroyed Penn State 27-0.

That was overwhelming proof that I should quit, so that's what I did. I wanted to do it with style. I waited till it was exactly 4 PM. Back then, we had a number you could call and get the exact time. So I called the time number, and at precisely 4 PM, I called in. I didn't ask for Percy. I just told them that I had decided to quit. I couldn't take it anymore. I then went and unplugged my phone so that they couldn't call me. I just sat on my couch and tried not to freak out. Carley woke up from a nap and walked into the living room. She looked at me and asked if I had quit. I just shook my head, yes. Lys had been laying down with Carley, and I took her and held her. She gave me a huge hug and all was better with my world.

Chapter 10

Looking back on it now, I wonder if quitting my job was the start of the downfall of our marriage. I quit my job in November, and it would be several months until I found another one. Before I quit, Carley would work as much or as little as she wanted. I worked all the time, and her income helped, but it wasn't necessary. Now it was our primary source of income, and she had to work as much as she could. I think the pressure got to her. She never really liked working. I loved working, and I became a workaholic. I loved being out and working with people and solving problems and being in charge. I had worked very hard to get where I was, and it was hard to give it up. I had a hard time adjusting to being the stay at home parent. I wasn't much of a cook, but I did clean. I also would do whatever I could for the kids.

I did love being a dad. I loved sitting on the couch with them and watching the stupid kid's shows they liked. While things were great with the kids, they were not with Carley and me. We started fighting about foolish crap all the time. She would complain about not having time to herself, and she felt trapped. She didn't like working so much. She wanted to be able to go out and have fun. I reminded her that she was only working 40 hours a week. I had been working double that or more. I had been looking for a job, but not everyone will give a chance to a disabled person. I was bringing in some money, but it wasn't much. Things slowly slid downhill. No matter what I did to try and save things, Carley seemed disinterested. She kept saying she felt trapped and just needed freedom.

In the spring, I knew the end was near if things didn't change. She kept using the phone and going into her bathroom and locking the door. She would stay there for hours. I started seeing the same number pop up on our caller ID. It was a Christian radio station. I asked Carley why a radio station kept calling our apartment. She lied about it a few times then admitted she had a friend that worked there. Later she admitted it was a guy, and his name was Deandre.

My heart broke because I knew what was going on. I knew that Carley was getting close to cheating on me if she hadn't already. I do believe men and women can be friends and not have sex. I do not think she can. I tried to talk to her and fix things, but it didn't work. She wouldn't speak to me about it. I did tell her I didn't like the fact that she was talking to this guy so much. She told me she was going to do what she wanted to do. She then told me she was going to out with him Saturday. I knew if she went out with him, she would cheat on me. I did try and talk her out of it. I told her if she wanted out, just tell me. All I asked was that she not cheat on me. When she came home, I knew she had sex with him. She couldn't look me in the eye. I was heartbroken, and there was nothing I could do to fix the situation.

I was desperate to try and fix my marriage. I talked Carley into going on a short weekend getaway, just the two of us. My mom watched the kids, and we took the train to Niagara Falls in Canada. We had a very romantic dinner in a revolving restaurant while the fireworks were going off. That view was incredible and will be something I will never forget. Even that couldn't help the marriage issues. Every time I talked to her, she would clam up and get angry. She kept telling me if I wanted things to work, I should just let her do whatever she wanted. I said that life doesn't work that way when you are married with two kids. She said that's how she wants her life to be. She also wanted to work less. She was growing more and more distant.

I decided to order Carley flowers for Mother's Day to show my appreciation for her being a good mother. I sent them to her at work because she had to work that day. I did not get the reaction I had anticipated. When she got home, she started one of the biggest fights we ever had. She was pissed that I spent our money on them because all they were going to do was die. A couple of times, she almost threw them at me. I didn't understand what her issue was. Come to find out right after they had delivered them Deandre showed up. He got upset with her, and that's why she was mad at me. I should have just filed for divorce. If she would fight like that over me buying her flowers, what was the point?

With my marriage falling apart, I knew I had to find another job fast. I finally got an excellent lead on a good job, and I was ecstatic. The company I was interviewing with was a contractor for General Motors. I was nervous about this interview. I wanted this job more than I had wanted any job. I realized I had a problem. The resume I had sent was incorrect. It stated I had a degree from Mott I didn't have. I was two classes short. I didn't know what to do. I made the snap decision just to fill out the application and keep up the lie for now.

The interview went great, and I took some pre-employment testing. They told me that I had done well. They would be in touch in a few days to schedule another interview. I was so excited about the interview. I felt like shit about lying. I knew the best thing would be just to call them up and confess. So that's what I did. I called them and explained the situation. I told them how bad I felt that I had lied. A few hours later, they called me back, and she said to me that they still wanted to go forward with the next interview.

When I went for my interview, I realized I had a big problem. I couldn't find the wheelchair accessible entrance. Generally, if you find the handicapped parking spaces, you can locate the path you need to take. Every door I saw had stairs at it. I drove around the building twice. I was about to be late for my interview. To make matters worse, I hate asking for help. But I knew I had to.

Finally, I saw someone walking into the building. I flagged them down and asked for help. I explained I was there for an interview, but I couldn't find an entrance suitable for a wheelchair. They didn't know either. They said security was just inside the door, and they would go in and ask. A couple of minutes later, a security guard came out and told me to drive down this huge ramp on the side of the building. I drove down there, and they opened a garage door. I pulled in and saw a ramp next to a handicapped space. I was a few minutes late, but she understood because of the circumstances. I had the interview, and I knew I knocked it out of the park. About a week later, they called and offered me the job which I happily accepted.

The job itself was perfect for me. I would be customer service for all the General Motors dealerships. I would help order parts or track shipments. I could check inventory and, if needed, call suppliers. There was a lot to learn and a lot of screens to know and how to get to them. Training for the job would be the first 30 days. After that, if we passed, we would listen to calls next to someone. Then they would sit next to us while we took calls. Then we would take our own calls. If we weren't taking our own calls after 60 days, they would fire us.

About 20 other people were starting with me. I just wanted to stand out and prove I was better than the rest. The training was a blast. I felt like I belonged with them. I made some friends and soon my friends, and I was the stars of the training class. The company also treated me better than any company ever had. They got me a garage door opener to get into the security garage to park. Let me tell you nothing beats parking in a heated parking garage during a Michigan winter. I didn't have to struggle with snow or anything. This job was excellent! At the end of the 30 day training period, my friend and I were the first two in the class to shadow another rep. A week later, I was taking calls on my own. The company assigned me to the southeast region, which meant most of the calls I took during the day were from that part of the country.

At home, things went from bad to worse. Carley decided to take a 2nd job. So suddenly the woman who didn't want to work one job now was excited about a 2nd one. This made no sense, and I knew something was up. After her first day of work, I knew the end was near. All she talked about was this guy she worked with Kyle. It was Kyle this and Kyle that and he was so awesome and on and on. I knew her, and I knew she would be replacing me with him when she got the nerve to do it. I decided with the help of my mom to start getting my ducks in a row. I couldn't take time off of work. I had to have my mom do a lot of legwork for me. She suggested I think about hiring an attorney. She wanted me to call one that my sister's ex-husband had used. The lawyer was excellent, and my mom was impressed with her. So on my lunch break, I called her office and talked to her over the phone. I was equally as impressed and hired her.

My mom paid her so Carley wouldn't wonder why money was missing. I wasn't ready to file just yet, but I was getting everything ready. In the meantime, Carley's behavior became more and more erratic. She would take the kids to daycare even on days she was not working. She would come home from work reeking of stale cigarette smoke. She claimed she was talking to people outside of work, and they were smoking. I knew better than that. I knew by now that everyone in Kyle's family smoked.

In July, Carley announced that the whole photography company was going on a four-day canoe trip. I was getting closer and closer to filing for divorce. When she came back from the canoe trip, she was even more distant. She was never home. She was always putting the kids in daycare. She would say she was working when I knew she wasn't. She wouldn't come home after work. She would claim she had to work late.

I stepped up the preparations to file for divorce. One of the problems I had was Carley had a family reunion. It was in Arkansas, and we had hotel reservations and everything. I had the OK from work to miss the days to go. By now, Carley knew that I knew she was cheating on me. She didn't care, and it certainly didn't stop her. Carley told me that I didn't have to go to her family reunion, but if I didn't go and act like the happy husband, she would just take Kyle. I was worried if she left the state with the kids, she may not come back. So I did what I thought I had to do. I called my attorney and told her to file everything. I couldn't go to her office, so she faxed the paperwork to me. I signed everything and faxed it back. She quickly filed everything and set out to serve Carley the paperwork.

I had no intention of going to the family reunion or letting Carley take the kids. I called my mom and had her pick up the kids from daycare. I knew Carley wasn't working, but if the kids were at daycare, that means she was out with Kyle. My mom ran to the apartment. Luckily we were scheduled to leave for the family reunion the following day. We all had suitcases packed. My mom just grabbed those and some other things I didn't want to leave there. I told my boss what was going on and she told me to leave.

I met my mom at the bank. I quickly opened another account and moved my money into my new account. I left Carley's money in the account we shared. We left to go to my grandparents' house to hide out while I figured out what to do next. Carley thought my mom had picked the kids up for her and would be dropping them off at the apartment. I wish I had been there to see her face when she realized that the kids' stuff was gone and I wasn't at work. I doubt she saw it coming. I am sure many will say what I did was mean.

Under the circumstances, what real choice did I have? We were hundreds of miles away before she knew what I had done. I needed a place to think and a place to hide out where we wouldn't be bothered. Carley may have guessed where we went, but she had only been there once. I doubt she could even remember the name of the city.

I was holding it together, barely in front of the kids. They knew something was wrong, but both were too young to understand what. The kids just knew we were going on a trip. I was an emotional wreck. I hadn't been sleeping or eating much recently. On the way to my grandparents, my mom did everything she could to get me to eat and to try and relax. I did call Carley and tell her I had the kids, and we were OK. We would be back in a few days. I needed time to think and get things figured out. Carley told me she called the police, but they wouldn't do anything. I refused to tell her where I was or where I was going. The last thing I needed was her trying to find us. I told her we would be back Sunday.

My aunt was at work at our apartment complex. I had her drive by, and she saw Kyle's car there. I knew Carley wasn't alone. I was pissed off. We were getting divorced, no matter what. When we finally arrived at my grandparents, they both met us as we pulled in. My grandmother gave me the biggest hug. I have to admit at that moment in time, and it was what I needed.

I just didn't understand why things had gone so wrong. Things changed when we got married for some reason. I was also feeling humiliated. I was ashamed by the fact that my marriage didn't even last a year. I went over and over in my head hundreds of times things I could have done differently. The simple fact was this. Marriage is a two-way street, and it takes two people working together to make it work. By no means am I perfect, and at times I could be challenging to live with. Noah had a lot of issues, and that added to the stress. But that did not make it OK for Carley to do what she did. Cheating on someone to me is the lowest of the low. Carley could have just left or told me she wanted a divorce, but instead, she lied and cheated.

Over the next few days, Carley and I talked a few times but got nowhere. She never really apologized. Carley was refusing to admit she had ever cheated on me. She kept insisting it was all in my head. That they were just friends, and she just enjoyed hanging out with him. I reminded her that is what she told Ronald about me, and we were sleeping together. Her past was against her on this. A few mutual friends had already told me the truth. But I didn't tell her that. Finally, after a very heated conversation, she admitted that she had cheated on me with a few people in the past six months. She wasn't that sorry about doing it. She wasn't happy, so she felt like that entitled her to do what she wanted. Carley wanted me to come home with the kids so we could work through things.

I agreed that I needed to come home and I told her I would be soon. I sure as hell deserved better. I was not going to continue to live like this. I didn't have to be married to be a dad. I was determined to be the best dad I could, regardless of if we were married or not. The kids were now going to be my main priority. I grew up without a dad, and I knew that Lys would not go through that. I loved Noah, and I was going to fight for him as much as I could. To me, he was my son, and that is all that mattered!

We headed home on Sunday. The drive is typically around 3 hours, but it seemed to take forever. The closer we got, the bigger the knots in my stomach got. I couldn't run and hide permanently. I had to face all this. The best way to do it would be to face it head-on. When we got home, Carley was there waiting for us. She came out and got the kids and gave them both hugs.

My mom was bringing in the stuff from the car. To her credit, she didn't say anything to Carley. I knew damn well she wanted to, but her silence was deafening. I did catch her, giving her the look of death a few times. I will admit I didn't view Carley the same way. I used to feel love when I looked at her. Now all I felt was anger and hatred. I hated her for what she did to our family and me! There just was no real reason for it. I am not perfect, and no one is, but I never abused her in any way. I was a good father to the kids, and I would never have cheated on her. Once my mom was gone, the real challenge began.

We started out talking calmly. I just really wanted answers as to why Carley would do this. I wondered what her thoughts were on everything. She said she wasn't happy, so she cheated on me. She felt trapped. She wanted the freedom to come and go when she wanted. I said this was stupid because she has two kids. You just can't go out and do what you want when you have two kids. I asked her if she would go to marriage counseling. She said no because they will tell her that she shouldn't cheat on me and she already knew that.

At this point, she offered me the stupidest thing I had ever heard. She wanted to stay married and just date other people from time to time. She said I could as well. All I could do when she said that was to shake my head and laugh. I then told her we were over, and she needed to get the hell out. I told her I was going forward with the divorce. We talked it out. She was going to live with Kyle at his dad's house. She would leave the kids with me. There wasn't room for them there.

Where Kyle lived was more of a party house and not suited for kids. I knew being a single dad to two kids wouldn't be easy. I loved them, and for their sake, I was willing to make sacrifices I needed to. This would also allow Carley to party as she wanted without dragging the kids along. All she was thinking about was her life and what she wanted in life. I knew she loved the kids, but she wanted her freedom more.

A couple of days later, Carley informed me that she had talked it over with her family. She would not be moving out and would not be leaving the kids with me. She was worried had she done that it would look bad on her. I was going to have to find a way out of this mess. The problem was anywhere I moved would need to be wheelchair accessible. And it isn't easy to find anything like that. Apartments have limited units. They filled quickly, and finding a house that I wouldn't have to rebuild is next to impossible. I checked on kicking Carley out, but her name was on the lease so that I couldn't do that. I was stuck with her.

At this point, the mere sight of her made me angry as hell. Now that everything was out in the open, Carley made no effort to hide what she was up to and was barely home. When she was home, she spent a lot of time on the phone to Kyle or god knows who else. The only thing keeping me going was the kids. Even the new job I loved was hard because I was very distracted. There were also a few times I would lose my composure at my desk. I was just under a lot of pressure. Between learning a new job and a home life that was a complete mess, I was barely functioning. I just knew I had to keep going. The kids needed me now more than ever.

Chapter 11

A few weeks after I filed for divorce, we had made plans to go to Cedar Point and visit Clem, who was working there. I was looking forward to this because I hadn't seen Clem since our wedding. Carley's good friend Amy would also be going with us. I had thought about canceling things or going by myself. Carley insisted on going, and for some reason, I relented and let her and Amy tag along. We would be staying at Clem's Friday and Saturday night and come home Sunday. I was hoping everything would go smoothly. There was part of me that wanted to shove Carley off the tallest ride and watch her fall. Clem had assured me he would bail me out of jail if I needed it. I highly doubt he was joking.

When we got to Clem's, we ordered pizza and talked. It was nice seeing him again. Since he moved to Ohio, we hadn't talked much in the past few years. We all played cards and just had a good evening. I did the best I could to try and forget everything and relax. That was much easier said than done. We left early the next morning for Cedar Point. We arrived just as the gates opened and started mapping out our plan for the day. Most rides we could go in the ride exit and skip the line. I could also ride everything twice without getting off. We could easily ride every ride we wanted to in just a few hours. We had plenty of time to walk around or catch a show. There was also a large hotel just off property that you could walk to that had a TGIFridays in it. That is where the girls wanted to eat dinner. That sounded like a great idea seeing I could never turn down a chance at a steak dinner.

We walked around a little bit and rode some rides. We were having a good time. For the first time in months, I felt myself relaxing. We rode everything that we wanted to twice. We decided to have an early dinner. We walked to the exit of the park that was next to the hotel. There was a small wait, so we decided to use the bathroom before dinner. When we came out of the bathroom, we saw Carley over by the front desk. She was talking to the front desk receptionist, which seemed a bit odd. Our table was ready. So we went in and sat down. Carley had with her some hotel pamphlets. I asked her why she had those. Carley told me that she and Kyle were planning to come down in a few weeks.

Hearing her say that to me honestly was like someone had punched me right in the stomach. I couldn't believe it. Clem said he could tell by my face that I was getting upset. The waitress came by, and I needed a drink. I ordered the largest long island ice tea they had. Carley was talking about maybe renting a room with a hot tub for her and Kyle. She went on and on about her upcoming trip with Kyle and how she liked spending time with him and his friends. Carley talked about how they always had a great time. The more she spoke, the madder I got. I remember almost being in tears with frustration. Clem and Amy just kept looking at her stunned, not knowing what to say or do. No one could believe what she was talking about right in front of me.

Thankfully the waitress arrived with my drink. This drink was huge, and it was damn good. I chugged it as fast as I could. It was gone in under five minutes, and I ordered another one. Clem and Amy both asked me to slow down, but neither of them could blame me. Carley was still going on and on. She even got up to use a payphone to call Kyle to tell him the information she had. My second drink came, and I drank that one a bit slower. When I was about half done with the second one, I kind of blacked out. To this day, I have no clue what I said or did once I blacked out. Next thing I knew, we were done eating. My second drink was empty, and Carley left the table quickly in tears. Clem and Amy decided we should split up to ease the tension.

Clem and I stayed at the table for a bit to let the girls get clear of us. I asked Clem what happened. I explained that I had no memory of anything after drinking half of my second drink. I don't even remember eating. Clem didn't give me specifics but explained it as me saying everything I had wanted to say for months.

He didn't blame me for anything. I did feel a lot less frustrated at this point. I wasn't sure if it was because of letting off some of the steam by telling Carley my real thoughts or because of the alcohol. I hadn't been this drunk in a long time, and it was well overdue. Clem and I just walked around and talked, which I needed more than anything. I had been holding too much in and living with all this day in and day out. I was also putting on the bravest face I could for the kids. I was exhausted. I didn't have many people I could count on. I knew I could tell Clem anything, and he would be there for me. This was one of the hardest times of my life.

We met back up with the girls, and I got a soda. I hoped that it would calm my stomach a bit. We went to a few of the shows and a small movie. They wanted to ride this roller coaster I hated called the Raptor. The reason I hated this thing is that all you did was spin and flip. Something that I didn't like. But the line was long. They needed me to ride so we could skip it. They talked me into it reluctantly.

I did not doubt that I would probably throw up. My goal was to make it through without dying. I believe you are upside down 18 times on the ride. Each one made me feel worse. After the first go-round, I was queasy, but they wanted a second ride. I just shook my head. I was afraid if I said anything I would throw up. By the end of the second go-round, it was all I could do to keep breathing. I didn't throw up, but I was as close as you could get. I needed off that damn ride and fast! I was concentrating on not getting sick. We decided to go. About half the way back to Clem's house, I made him pull over, and I did get sick.

When we got back to Clem's house, I went and laid down. That may have been the best night's sleep that I had gotten in months. Usually, I don't sleep well after drinking. I must have just been mentally and physically exhausted. I just passed out. I woke up well-rested but still stressed out about everything. I was ready to head back home. I had to work the following day. I knew it was going to be a long week seeing I was already exhausted.

My mom dropped the kids off before I got home. I hadn't seen the kids in a few days, and I did miss them. If it wasn't for them, I might never go home. I got home, and the kids ran up to me with hugs. Nothing is better than hugs and kisses from your kids. We had dinner and then gave the kids the presents we had bought them. We bought them some stuffed animals and other toys.

One of the things we bought Noah was a plush bank that looked like Snoopy's dog house. It was adorable, and he loved it. He went and put all the change he could find in it. I loved seeing them so happy and smiling. I was anxious about how the divorce would be on them. Right now, Noah was old enough to know that something was going on. My goal was to make it as easy on them as possible. I would try and protect them as much as I could. After dinner, Carley said she needed to go to the store and get milk. I knew this was bull shit. She was just using that as an excuse to see Kyle. I am not even sure why she lied at this point. The funny thing was we lived 10 minutes at the most from the grocery store. She would be gone three hours and come back reeking of cigarette smoke. Carley wasn't even smart enough to go to the store and buy what she went for. The number of times she came back empty-handed was comical. I was sick of the sight of her.

A few days later, I came home from work, and Carley told me she had to go to the store. As soon as she left, Noah came up to me and said he had a secret. My heart sank. I already knew what it was, but I wanted him to tell me anyway. Noah said that his mother told him not to tell me, but he had to say something. He said that his mother's new friend came over and spent the day there while I was at work. This made me about as angry as I could ever get.

I was doing my best to keep the kids out of it. Now she is parading her new boyfriend around them and in my home no less. Usually, I am not an angry or violent person. Whenever I get close to losing it, I always thought back to when I was younger. One memory that has still stuck with me was one time Dick started hitting Kayla and me. My mother laid over us to shield us. It has always been a powerful memory. I never want my kids to witness such a thing. I could typically never imagine myself being violent to Carley or the kids. I will never understand the people that parent through fear. It just doesn't make any damn sense to me. But in this exact moment, I was seething with anger a capable of anything I had finally snapped.

When Carley got back a little while later the fight started right away, I don't even think I let her shut the front door. I sent the kids into their room, and we were off. She tried to get to our room and shut the door. I got there before her. She admitted Kyle had been there, and she said she was going to do whatever she wanted. She didn't give a damn what I thought. I grabbed her with both hands, and Carley tried to pull away. In my angry state, she wasn't getting away. I can't even remember what I was thinking at this point. All I knew was I was pissed, and I have had enough!

Just then, there was a knock at the door, and the doorbell rang. It startled me back to my senses, and I let Carley go. She went and answered the door, and it was my uncle. He said he was just driving by and stopped by to check on me. He took one look at me and got me out of there. We went out to a local bar. I started drinking and just talking about what had been going on. My uncle had gone through a divorce the year before. He understood a lot of what I was going through. And after a few drinks, I felt much better.

I was ashamed for putting my hands on Carley and letting my anger get the best of me. I shudder to think what would have happened had my uncle not shown up. It wasn't something he ever did before or since. I had a guardian angel looking out for me that night. I was capable of anything at that moment. When I got home a few hours later, I was a bit drunk. I talked with Carley. I did apologize for getting physical. I felt terrible, and I shouldn't have done it. I made it clear had she did not have Kyle around the kids, and it wouldn't have happened. I made it clear that it was not OK. I expected her to uphold her agreement. She said she would, and I didn't believe a damn word she said.

Carley's behavior was the least of my concerns. Lys hadn't been feeling well for some reason. She kept throwing up after eating or drinking and choking. Other than that, she acted fine. We thought it was the flu. We had talked, and both agreed that if she kept doing it, we would take her to the doctor. I was at work, and my mom called. She said that our sitter had called her and Lys was acting strange. She had chocked a couple of times. She was going to pick her up and take her to the doctor. I thanked her and gave her permission and told her to keep me posted. My mom said she couldn't get her into our doctor. She was going to take her to the emergency room.

This little girl was my life, and she was about the only bright spot I had. I had worked for the rest of my day and headed home. I had called Carley to tell her what was going on. We were going to meet up at home then head up to the emergency room. I had just gotten through the door when my mom called. She said we had to get up to the hospital right away; it was an emergency. They had checked Lys all over and weren't sure what was wrong. They decided to do an x-ray to see if they could find anything. Just after they took the x-ray, they came in and asked if Lys was wearing a necklace. My mom said no, why? They showed her the film, which showed a small metal object in her throat.

. They were going to prep her for emergency surgery, but we had to get there. I started freaking out, and I screamed at Carley we had to go. She asked me what was going on. I tried the best I could to explain. We were 30 minutes from the hospital, and we had to go. She said she had to make a call. I grabbed the phone and whipped it across the room. Then I shoved her out the door. My only priority at that point was to get to my baby.

I didn't give a damn what the speed limit was. I went as fast as I could. We were there in no time. When we got there, they had Lys in a room. They were doing everything they could to keep her still. They were pretty sure the object lodged in her throat was a penny. The doctor said had it gotten stuck at any other angle, she would have died. We were fortunate that she was able to breathe. They were still concerned that if it moved even the smallest amount, she could choke to death.

This was one of the scariest moments of my life. I felt so helpless! I would have done anything to change places with her. I also felt so bad for not doing something sooner. I had no clue it was this serious. It is just one of those moments as a parent; you just beat yourself up over. The more we tried to keep her still, the more she fought us. Finally, they decided to give her an IV to give her fluids. They would also provide her with something to calm her down a bit.

We sat and started talking to figure out how all this happened. When we went to Cedar Point, we bought Noah the plush Snoopy bank. He instantly put change in it. The problem was that when you shook it, the change came flying out. We tried to fix it but ended up just taking the money out of it. Lys had a bad habit as most kids do of putting everything in her mouth. We think we missed a penny when we picked up the money, and she found it and swallowed it. We were so lucky she hadn't chocked to death. We got lectured by the nurses and the doctor to be more careful. Carley wanted to argue back, but I understood that it is their job. I was feeling like the worst parent in the world. I just wanted my baby to get better.

Carley was pissing me off while we were at the hospital. She kept disappearing over and over to use the phone. She claimed to be calling her family. I knew damn well it was Kyle. I was getting so frustrated with her. Our baby is lying in a hospital bed, getting ready for surgery, and her mother was calling her boyfriend. I was trying not to get angry, but that was becoming increasingly difficult. Today was Friday, and Lys would have surgery then stay in the hospital for a few days. They would go down with a small tweezer-like instrument and pull the penny out. If it wouldn't come out, then they would look at more invasive surgery. The hope was that it wouldn't be needed. When they put the IV in Lys's little arm, they didn't numb it enough, and she cried as hard as I have ever heard her. My heart broke into a million pieces. I felt so helpless. I always view my job as protecting her and keeping her safe. I could do nothing to help her.

They were able to get the penny out, although it had started to rust. There were marks in her throat where it had been rubbing. It was near midnight when Lys got back to her room. They did tell us when she was released. We would have to watch her closely for a day or two. She would need as much rest as possible. We would have to watch what she ate and drank in case of potential issues. They seemed to think after a short recovery time; she would be fine. They even gave us the penny as a kind of souvenir, and it is in her baby book. With Lys being so little and being scared, my mom offered to stay with her the first night. We would come up and relieve her first thing in the morning. Regardless of who was with her, it was going to be a long night!

Once we got home, the fight started. It didn't help I was already exhausted from working all day and then being at the hospital all night. I had been up for about 20 hours. I was beyond frustrated with everything. Carley seemed more worried about her Cedar Point trip with Kyle than Lys. They wanted to leave early Monday morning. Carley asked if she could still go. I said I didn't want her to go. Someone would need to be home with Lys, and I had to work.

I asked her why she can't reschedule it. She said ten people were going. I wondered if she and Kyle could go on a different day. I was so angry that we even had this fight. Our daughter was lying in a hospital bed that very minute. Her mother was more worried about her vacation. I just went to bed and tried to sleep although I didn't get much sleep. We got up and ready at sunrise. We headed back up to the hospital as soon as we could.

Once we got to the hospital, I was relieved to see Lys up already. She instantly smiled when she saw us and gave us hugs. That made me feel so much better. I knew she was not out of the woods just yet, but she seemed to be her old self. My mom looked a bit beat up. I doubt she had slept much at all. She could tell by the look on my face I wasn't exactly thrilled about something. Carley left the room for one of her phone calls. I filled mom in on what was going on. She said she had a follow up with her cancer doctor on Monday that she couldn't miss. She would watch Lys on Tuesday if I needed it. I told her thanks, and I would keep her posted. Then I sent her home. She would be up later once she got a nap and a shower.

This was going to be a long day. Our main objective was to try and keep Lys as stationary as possible. One minute she would be coloring, and the next she would be trying to jump on the bed. She also had to be careful because she still had her IV in. They didn't plan on taking that out till Sunday. My mom came back early in the evening. Carley and I went to get something to eat. While we ate, we got into a fight about her damn Cedar Point trip again. I told her my mother couldn't watch Lys, and the doctors had advised we keep her home.

I wasn't supposed to miss a day in my first ninety days. This would be my second one. I wasn't sure what work would do. Carley said she would have her mom or aunt watch her, but they wouldn't do it at our place. I didn't like that idea at all. She needed to be home. The doctor said to keep her home, and that is what was going to happen. I was so sick of this fight by now. To me, it should have been simple. I had to work, and she didn't. It really shouldn't have been that hard to put your daughter first. I was sorry her plans had to change. That is what happens when you're a parent. She wanted me to tell her it was OK to go, and I wouldn't do it. By now, I damn well knew she would go. I would do what I had to for my daughter.

That night my mom couldn't stay with Lys. The night before had taken a lot out of her. So it was either going to be Carley or I staying with Lys. Carley said she would, but I didn't trust her, so we both stayed with her. They had a chair that folded out for Carley to lay in. I had to stay in my wheelchair, and there is no way to sleep in that. When the sun came up, I was beyond ready to get home. They took the IV out and gave us a prescription for an antibiotic.

They were still a bit concerned and told us to keep a very close eye on her. We packed up and headed home. I was glad that my baby was OK. She was happy to be home and especially to have the IV out. It wasn't long after we got home, and the fighting started again. Carley would not let the Cedar Point trip go. She said it was unfair of me to try and get the entire group to cancel plans. To be clear, I wasn't telling the whole group they shouldn't go. I was just telling her. I was only telling her that because our child was sick and I had to work. Had I not had to work, I would have let her go. Hell, I wanted her to go so I could have a couple of days with no fighting.

Carley woke me up early the next morning to tell me she was leaving. She begged me not to lock her out. I couldn't have kicked her out had I wanted to. I had already checked. When she left, I went and got Lys and took her into my room to cuddle with her. I loved to watch her sleep. She was such a little sweetheart and had stolen my heart. I made a mental list of all I had to do that day. I knew I would have to call my boss. I did love this job, and I hated risking it, but Lys needed me. I never gave it a second thought.

I had gone back to sleep for a few hours but woke up before I was supposed to be at work and called my boss. All I got was her voicemail. I left my number and then went through everything about Lys that had happened over the weekend. I told her I had doctor's notes and everything to prove what had happened. I explained that Lys couldn't go to daycare. I had no choice but to stay home with her. I didn't tell her anything about Carley, but she knew all about my divorce. I waited for her to call me back, but she never did. I also called my lawyer and filled her in on everything. Then I called my mom to tell her what had been going on. She said she would come in on Tuesday and watch the kids till either I got home or Carley did. This was a mess, and I just wanted to get through it.

The rest of the day was excellent. The kids were playing like normal, and Lys was acting as if nothing had happened. She was running around and just being her usual giggly self. I was delighted to see that. I kept asking if her throat hurt and she said no. It certainly hadn't hurt her appetite at all. She was eating as much as I would let her. I was careful about what I gave her. We all sat on the couch and watched some movies and cuddled together. I didn't miss the constant fighting with Carley. This was a precursor to what single fatherhood would be daily. I wasn't complaining one bit!

That night I had slept better than I had in a while. I woke up refreshed and ready to go. I got ready for work. Just as I was about ready, my mom came in. We talked for a bit, and I thanked her for saving me. I filled her in on how Lys was doing and that everything seemed OK. I left for work and was fine till I got to my desk. That is when the nerves hit. I became worried about everything. Several of my coworkers came over to check on me. They were shocked when I told them about Lys and glad to know she was OK. My boss came up a little while after I got there. She asked how Lys was doing right away. She said she could tell by the tone in my voice that I was worried. She said I had nothing to worry about job-wise.

Chapter 12

I was relieved to know my job was safe. This job was going well. The company kept coming up to me, trying to figure things out to help me and make things easier. Soon I was one of the top reps in the office. The big boss once joked with me he could tell when I was on a break because the number of calls holding went up. That made me feel awesome. Especially after everything I had dealt with because of Percy. He destroyed my self-confidence. My personal life may have been in shambles, but for once, my work life was on point.

Carley ended up moving out around Thanksgiving. The hardest part was dividing up everything. We didn't have much, but what we did have we tried to split evenly. Carley kept anything she, or her family bought, and so did I. Unfortunately for me, Carley and her family had purchased a lot of our furniture. I was going to have to get a lot of stuff and fast. I got bunk beds for the kids as well as a kitchen table and chairs. They wouldn't be able to deliver them for a few days after Carley moved out. Carley and I had also agreed on a temporary custody agreement for both kids. We decided to share custody for both kids, and we would switch every Sunday. Legally I had no rights to Noah, but Carley assured me she would still let me see him. Many people told us it was a dumb arrangement. I thought we could pull it off. I had to be more than every other weekend type of father. I made that promise to Lys when she was born, and I meant it!

The day Carley moved out, I had to work. I certainly didn't trust her there unsupervised, so my mom said she would keep an eye on her. I only got about ten phone calls at work with them screaming at each other. I fully expected to have the police called a couple of times, but we didn't get that far. My aunt made sure all the locks were changed, and I had a new lease. In case things didn't work with Kyle, Carley had no right to move back in. The kids could have, but Carley never would live with me again.

I dreaded going home that night. When I got home the only furniture I had was a TV. The apartment just felt empty and sad. I cried a lot that night. I am not sure if it was because my marriage was over or relief that I wouldn't have to put up with all the bull shit anymore. Maybe a combination of the two. I was now a single father of two. Things got better once we got furniture and slowly but surely I started piecing my new life together.

When I had the kids, I was excellent, and they kept me busy and happy. However, the day arrived when I had to take the kids to Carley. They would be there for a week. I had never lived alone. It didn't take long for the depression to set in. I tried to keep myself as busy as possible. I talked on the phone a lot and spent obscene amounts of time on the internet. I had issues sleeping. No matter what I tried, I was only getting four hours of sleep of a night. The time that scared me the most was when I was driving to work. I remember staring at a concrete pillar on the expressway and just thinking I should floor it and turn left and plow right into the pillar and end it all. I had that same thought several days in a row. The only thing that stopped me was the kids. I knew they were counting on me. I couldn't leave them without their dad.

I knew I needed to find happiness in something other than the kids. Thankfully work was going well, and that helped. I was now in charge of a few projects. I was also helping train new employees. I loved passing on all the little tricks I had picked up along the way. I had gotten a nice raise and a new boss. His name was Dan. He was great at pointing out little things I needed to change. He said I was on my way to being a supervisor someday. He wanted me to learn as much as I could.

Around this time, promotions were becoming available. Several of them I thought I had a shot at, but I didn't end up getting them. I wanted to know why so I talked with my boss Dan. The main reason I didn't get promoted was that I didn't have my degree. That would always hamper me moving forward. Someone with a degree will always have a leg up when it comes to raises and promotions.

Dan asked me how far away I was from a degree. I told him just a few classes. He pointed out that our company had tuition reimbursement. He said the program was perfect for me. I asked for the information. I checked into going to the University of Michigan Flint. I was worried about Lys, and both Carley and my mom said they would help me. I applied to U of M Flint, and I was accepted. I then applied for the tuition reimbursement program. They accepted me as well. Most of my credits from Mott transferred. I was all set to begin classes in the fall.

I would have to pay for the classes then submit proof I paid for them. They would pay me back. If I didn't pass the classes, I would then have to pay the company back. I submitted all the paperwork, but I never heard from them. I was starting to freak out. I didn't have the money for the classes and books. I only did it because I knew the company would be paying me back.

I went and talked to Dan because no one was answering me. He thought he had talked to me about it already. Dan said that he had received an email a month before advising him to tell me that they had changed the rules for the tuition reimbursement program. Only one person per department was eligible, and someone else got it from my department. The only way I could afford to do this was with the tuition reimbursement program. I would never have done it without knowing they would pay me back. I know rules change. But why didn't they tell me? I had a huge mess, and I had no clue what I was going to do. It was too late to back out of the classes. Luckily I was able to get a student loan to cover it, but I would still have to pay that back.

Because my life wasn't complicated enough, I decided to try dating. I decided to try online dating for the first time. The first woman that I got serious with after Carley was named Kristen. She was pretty with red curly hair. She didn't give a damn about me being in a wheelchair. I fell too hard and too fast. I think in part because I wanted to prove I could move on just like Carley had done. Kristen and I would talk all the time. We emailed all day while we were at work.

We met up, and she introduced me to her family. I enjoyed spending time with Kristen and her family. It didn't take long for her faults to start showing. If my attention was not entirely on her all the time, she would get pissed and start yelling. If I talked to the kids while I was on the phone with her, we got in a fight. When I was at work, if I didn't respond fast enough, we got in a fight. I had two small kids they needed me to. I had made it clear to her from the start that she would never be number one. That spot was for the kids. Finally, I just couldn't do it, and I broke things off with her. I was not going to let anyone come between me and the kids.

The weeks I didn't have the kids, I still very much wanted to see them whenever possible. I would arrange my work schedule so I could get out earlier. I would drive across town and pick them up from daycare. Then I would drive to Carley's work and wait with them till she got off work. I didn't get much time with them. That few minutes meant the world to me. I would make sure to get a hug and a kiss. The apartment still felt quiet and lonely. I was still a long way from where I needed to be mentally, but I was moving in the right direction.

Eventually, a few months later, I tried online dating again. I met Holly. We seemed to hit it off right away. She worked third shift but could chat online while at work. We would talk about everything and nothing for hours. I still wasn't sleeping much, so being up all night talking wasn't hard to do. She was a single mother with a daughter around Lys's age. The only problem was she lived over an hour away. The more time I spent talking with her, the more I liked her. She made it clear the feelings were mutual.

I managed to screw it up completely. I didn't hear from Holly for a few days. I started thinking she was cheating on me. In reality, I made her pay for things that weren't her fault. I had never taken the time to deal with the emotional baggage Carley had given me. Once things calmed down, we talked, but there was no recovery from all the damage I did. I knew I had to take a break and heal from everything that had happened. Otherwise, I would drag along all the emotional baggage into every relationship.

Carley and I had the important things agreed to for the divorce. We were still fighting over some of the finer details. We had a settlement conference in my attorney's office with Carley and her attorney. Carley tried to play hardball with me, and it failed miserably. They wanted to go to court and fight for custody. She was going to try and claim because of my disability I was unable to care for Lys. A few things were really against her in this argument. For one, I was already taking care of her on my own. And another was one of the judges happens to also be in a wheelchair, so the plan of attack wouldn't have sat well with him.

My attorney looked at Carley; she planned to pull every skeleton she had in her closet out and show it to everyone. The look on Carley's face was priceless. She even started to cry. I have to admit I found that moment very satisfying. I didn't want to mud sling, but I would do what I had to. Carley and her attorney stormed out. A few weeks later, Carley called me and said she wanted the divorce to be over. She wanted to know what it would take just to settle everything. I wrote out everything and gave her my list. Much to my surprise, she agreed to everything. We would switch custody every other week as we had been. We would alternate holidays, and she decided not to seek child support.

We went to court and signed the papers, and we were officially divorced. The hardest part was really, no matter what happened. I had to deal with Carley for the rest of my life. I had better suck it up and learn to put things behind me. There are times when I was angry and frustrated. But the most important thing for me is to be a dad. I couldn't let my frustration with Carley get in the way of that.

I was relieved to now have my divorce final. Work, however, had become frustrating. I was still mad about the tuition reimbursement mess. One of the ladies on my team Allie was talking about quitting and going to work for a local phone company. They were looking to add people, and they were paying well. Allie asked for a copy of my resume. I didn't think anything about it again till they called me. I said no at first, but they were persistent.

Eventually, I did agree just to come in and talk. I took a half-day off of work and went in to see what the company had to say. The sales pitch they gave me about the future and the company vision was impressive. By the time I left the interview, I was thinking about it. I also knew I loved my job and leaving a place I loved, and that loved me was very risky. Had it not been for the tuition reimbursement program issues, I would never have even talked to them. I should have just spoken to Dan and admitted I was upset. But that is not what I did, and I don't know why. My only guess would be the male ego, which leads to more trouble than its worth.

About a week later, Dan pulled me into a private meeting. The phone company had called him. He was not happy, and I didn't blame him. He wanted to know if I was seriously thinking about leaving. I lied and said no. I admitted that I had met with them. I lied and said I wasn't considering it. He knew I was disappointed about not getting a promotion. He said the company was looking at ways to open up more opportunities for me. They were looking at ways to work around my disability. This should have ended all my talk with the phone company. Outside of the tuition issue, the company and the job had been fantastic. I now realize they respected me more than I thought they did.

The director of the phone company called and wanted to talk to me personally. I said for me to leave, I needed more money. She asked how much and I just threw a dollar an hour more than they offered. I thought that would be the end of it. I was wrong, and a couple of hours later, she called back and said we had a deal. I accepted the job and was suddenly scared to death that I had just screwed up royally.

The training class was for ten people. I was the only guy outside of the lead trainer. His name was Art, and we hit it off instantly. The new job was in customer service. There was a lot to learn as far as telecommunications and how it all worked. My main job would be to take calls from residential customers and answer billing questions or handle complaints. I would also be setting up a new service and running credit reports. It helped that I had taken calls in the call center before. Allie had started a few weeks before I did, so it was nice to know someone there.

When I worked for GM, the system was excellent and up to date and modern. I expected that with the phone company. What I found was vastly different. Their system was old and slow. Had I been able to go crawling back, I would have, and I wanted to. I had to make this work, but I was not thrilled about it. This had nothing to do with the phone company. They were great and were treating me well. This had more to do with me making a mistake. And it did affect my job performance. I was not happy about work, and I wasn't happy about my personal life. Then Carley called me up about halfway through my classes and told me she would not watch Lys for me. My mom was having health issues so that she couldn't do it either. So there went school. My life was a total mess, and a lot of it was because of my stupid decisions.

Chapter 13

The first few months of being a single dad were complicated. I loved being a dad, but as a single dad, it was a lot of work. We found out Noah had special needs. Doctors diagnosed him with Asperger's Autism. I had to get myself up and ready in the morning then get Noah up. I never knew if he would get ready without a meltdown. Sometimes he was great, and sometimes getting out the door was a fight. I would then get Lys up and dressed. Then get everyone loaded into my truck and drive over to where Carley was living. Honestly, there were days when I was exhausted by the time I got to work. When Noah had terrible mornings, it could take an extra 30 minutes or more. There were times he would crawl underneath the kitchen table where I couldn't get him. Or he would hide in his room not wanting to come out. I couldn't fit my chair into his room to get him.

I feel horrible admitting this, but at times when he was under the table, I would pull him out by whatever I could grab. Those were the mornings I would get so frustrated with him. I know I didn't handle it right. I feel guilty even now for having done that. The whole time all this was going on, the clock in my head is ticking. I knew I am going to be late for work. Thankfully I had a boss who understood what was going on. My boss wasn't happy. I was late, but they worked with me. I was very thankful for their understanding. After work, I would pick the kids up with their sitter and go home and make dinner. Then I would help Noah with any homework, which may or may not come with another meltdown.

One of the problems we were having with Asperger's Autism is they don't handle change well. They need consistency, and Noah didn't have that. He was going back and forth every week. Carley's house didn't have a set of stable rules, or a set bedtime mine did. If he didn't want to get up and go to school when he was with Carley, she wouldn't fight with him about it. At my house, I didn't give a damn how much he fought and argued. He was still going to school.

Lys would kind of a go with the flow as far as the change. She would be fine after a day or two. Noah wouldn't be OK for four or five days. By the time he adjusted to being with me, it would be time to send him back to his mother's house. My frustration with how he was acting was through the roof. I just didn't know what to do. I had him retested by another expert. They came back with the same results. That meant now we had two separate tests by two different experts, all saying the same thing. Carley didn't agree with the diagnosis. She was going to get him retested. I have no clue why she didn't agree with the doctors.

Noah's school called me for a meeting to discuss everything going on with him. We had to try and figure out a plan on what to do. Carley had known about the conference for weeks but never told me. I doubted she wanted me there. I made arrangements to take a few hours off work to go. I never told Carley the school invited me. I thought it would be a pleasant surprise. One of the topics was an incident that happened a few weeks before. Kyle had dropped Noah off to school and left. The only problem was there was no school. The teachers were there for a work day but all students had the day off. When the school tried to call Carley, she never answered and never called them back. They called me at work, but I couldn't leave. It took me a couple of hours to get a hold of anyone who could go pick him up.

The school also wasn't happy with his attendance. Every week Carley had him; he missed 2-3 days. He would interrupt the teacher and was just a pain in the ass. I mentioned the diagnosis he had received twice. The school had no clue what I was talking about. Carley had not shown them any paperwork or even mentioned it to them. They had known we wanted to get him tested but were unaware that we had done it.

I brought my paperwork and gave it to them. Carley shot me a dirty look and informed the school she believed doctors had misdiagnosed him. All I could do was shake my head. I know all too well, it's not easy to raise a special needs child. Carley refused to do anything. She wanted an easy road. The school said they would need to go over the testing results. We would have another meeting in a few weeks.

A few days later I got a call from the school. They had received a letter from Carley's lawyer saying the school was no longer allowed to call me about Noah. I also got a cease and desist letter in the mail. The latter said I had to turn over all school and medical records that I had for Noah. It also noted that my mom nor I were allowed to seek any medical treatment for him. If I didn't stop doing what I was doing, they would try to have me thrown in jail. I called my attorney, and she said she had gotten the letter as well, and I had to comply with it. All I wanted was the best for him.

One day at work, my phone rang, and it was my mom. One minute later, Carley called and left a message. My heart sank! You know its bad news when your mom and your ex-wife call you a minute apart. I even made a joke about it to my coworkers, who all agreed it can't be good. My mom had the kids up and ready when Noah had a meltdown. He did not want to go to school. As she was fighting with him, Carley showed up to drop something off. She said if Noah didn't want to go to school, then he didn't have to. My mom said he was going like it or not. They started fighting, at which point Carley pushed my mom, and she fell. My mom got back up and decked Carley, and she fell. Carley grabbed Noah, and they left.

Carley claimed that my mom hit her first. She did admit to pushing my mom, but only after my mom had hit her. I talked to both kids separately. They both said Carley pushed grandma first. I think it's safe to say that my mom's version was correct. That was when Carley informed me that Noah would no longer be staying with me. She promised me that I could still see him every other weekend.

We tried every other weekend for a couple of months. Noah's behavior during the weekend was horrible. I still had my rules, and I expected him to follow them. I was supposed to pick him up Carley called me and said not to bother. She told me that Noah didn't want to come over. He said I was mean to him. I guess I was if you're going to call making him behave mean. I couldn't let him do whatever he wanted and then expect Lys to follow the rules. She would have started acting just like him, and I couldn't have that.

There was a heartbreaking moment a few months later. Carley had taken the kids trick or treating. I was following along in my truck because it was freezing out. Noah had gotten cold, so he joined me in the truck. This was the first time we had been able to talk since everything happened. He asked me if I was his real dad. Carley hadn't taken the time to explain to him that I wasn't his real dad. He told me that he thought I was, and I just didn't love him anymore. I started to tear up.

I was so angry! I knew how that felt. I would never do that to him. Even if I had divorced his mother, I would never have taken it out on Noah. I tried to make another agreement with Carley, but she refused. I told her she needed to talk to Noah about everything. She said she would, but I didn't trust her. She said that she was thinking about trying to find Noah's real dad. He had been paying child support for years but had never met him. Noah deserved so much better than what was going on. After this, I never really saw Noah again. She refused to let me see him. The whole situation broke my heart.

Unfortunately, work was just as chaotic as my personal life. The phone company I was working for announced they decided to close our office. I did get some possibly good news. I had heard from friends that GM had lost the contract for my old job. The new company would be hiring new representatives. I applied, and within days I got a call for an interview. I got called back for another interview. Then they called all my references. They told me they would call in a few days. I thought for sure I had it. But I never got the call.

I asked a few people if they could find out what happened. A few days later, one of my friends called. She told me that they were all set to hire me back. Dan advised them not to. He said that all I would do is work there till I found a better paying job. I wish I had reached out and talked to him. I owed him the truth because he was one of the best bosses I ever had. I wish some things would have ended up different.

The good thing about being laid off was I was home when Lys started school. Lys wasn't ready to start school when she turned five. She was behind the other kids. She was falling behind and becoming frustrated. We decided to put her in a slower-paced class for her first year and hold her back. They figured she would be fine after that. I still remember how cute she was on her first day. The funny part was her book bag was bigger than she was. She fell backward once because it was so heavy. She wasn't hurt because she landed on her book bag. She looked like a turtle on its back as she tried to get up.

I loved helping out in her classroom when I could. I was worried about how the kids would handle me being in a wheelchair. The kids didn't care about that. I loved all the holiday parties and helping them with their crafts. Whenever I helped another kid with their project, Lys would always want to be right next to me. She made sure they knew I was her dad. She would let me help anyone, but she was marking her territory.

Times like that showed me that I was as important to her as she was to me. Sometimes it's the small things you do that mean the most. We didn't have a lot of money, and I couldn't spoil her like I wanted to. But those things aren't as important as the time I spent with her. Some of my favorite memories with her at this age was when we would lay on the couch together. We would watch her shows or a movie she picked out.

After being out of work for over a year, I finally got an excellent lead. I had applied to one of the world's largest telecommunications companies. I found it a little odd that one of the prerequisites for the job was sales experience. I didn't have much in the way of sales experience. Then I remembered my experience of selling sports memorabilia. I did it as a hobby, but I did manage to make some extra money doing it. Thankfully that sales experience was enough to pass the phone interview. The next level was a face to face interview and a computer test. The test began, and it was pretty easy. After the examination, we were all told that everyone had passed. The final step would be an interview with a manager and the department director. They had many dates and times available, but I decided to take one that day. The reason being is it was almost an hour away from home, and it made sense to get it done on the same day.

My interviewers' name was Kathy, and she seemed very pleasant and friendly. The office was on the 3rd floor, so we took the elevator up to the office. We went to one of the back conference rooms. Kathy began the interview by outlaying what the job entailed and what the company's expectations would be. I knew when I started the interview process that the job would entitle sales. The more Kathy talked, the more apparent it became that sales would be the top priority.

Kathy asked me about my sales experience. I again relied on my sports collectibles business. I explained I had to be an excellent salesman and build quick chemistry with my customers. I talked at length about my previous job with the smaller phone company. I told her I understood telecommunications terminology and how it worked. I talked a lot about their internet product and how businesses could benefit from it. When I started talking about the internet, she got a massive smile on her face. I knew I had passed the interview. She said that they were always an equal opportunity employer and prided themselves on being accommodating.

They called the next day and said the last step would be a urine test. Oddly enough, the urine test scared me more than anything. It wasn't for reasons that you may think. I wasn't a drinker, and I haven't done any illegal drugs. It's almost impossible to pee in a cup when you are in a wheelchair. If I try and stand up, I need one hand to balance, and that leaves me just one hand to do everything else. If I got pee all over me in the process, then that is what I had to do. To make sure I would have to go when I got there I drank a lot of water before I went to bed. I knew I wouldn't go to the bathroom until the test. When I woke up that morning, I was very nervous and very uncomfortable.

I was starting to get annoyed. They had called everyone that came before me and several that arrived after me. I was ready to burst. My mom, who drove me, went up to see what was taking so long. They told me that they had no testing rooms for anyone in a wheelchair. None of the rooms had bars in it. They weren't even sure if my chair would fit in the rooms. After talking things over, they decided to bend the rules. They allowed my mother to help me. Thankfully their back up plan worked although it was a tad embarrassing. At least it was done.

A few days after I took the test they called and offered me the job! I would be making more money than I ever had in my life. I felt like a huge weight lifted off my shoulders. I admit I was the happiest I had been in a while. I wouldn't have to worry about bills or if we would have enough food anymore. Unless you have dealt with that, you really will never understand all the stress you feel.

The first call I made was to my mom. I don't think I would have ever made it through the past year without her. I was about to begin a brand new adventure. For the first time in a long time, I was very excited about my future. I had a great job with one of the largest companies in the world. I was also going to be part of a union for the first time. I knew I would have to work hard, but that was second nature. I have never been afraid to prove myself. I was also excited by the career possibilities.

The drawbacks were that the job was an hour away. The commute would be rough, especially in winter. I talked it over with my mom. We came up with a plan for Lys. On my weeks with Lys, my mom would come in on Monday and get Lys to school. She would keep her all week, and I would get her back on Friday. I hated doing this but having my mom come and get her every morning would be rough on everyone.

One thing I started doing on Wednesdays with Lys. I would pick her up, and we would have daddy/daughter date night. We would go to our favorite restaurant for a kid's night. They had a clown, games, face painting, and food specials for families. We both looked forward to date night. One piece of advice to other fathers is to date your daughters. I am not talking about anything creepy. What I mean is to go out and show your daughters you love them. Even if you don't have the money go to a park or a library, take them out and get some alone time. Talk to them. Listen to their stories. Let them know how much they mean to you. Let them know they can count on you. Because if you don't show them, then someone else will.

As much as I knew, I would miss being a full-time dad. I was excited to start a new job. I really couldn't even sleep the night before my first day. I was very nervous about meeting my coworkers. When people first meet me, my disability usually throws people off. Especially if they didn't have experience with a disabled person, if you put me in a room of strangers, I can usually tell who in the room has dealt with a disabled person before. Someone who has experience with a disabled person will treat them just like everyone else. People who have not to tend just to stand, stare, and not say anything. You can just tell by their facial expressions they are very uncomfortable.

I arrived at the office almost an hour before I needed to be there. I knew it would be crucial for me to make a great first impression. Companies tend to see more of what you can't do than what you can. It had been a long year, and I was going to fight as hard as I could. Little did I know then it would take everything I had to survive. This job would fight and challenge me in ways I had never dreamed of.

I realized it was time to get out of the van when I saw a group of people gathering near the door. You could also tell that everyone was very nervous. I rolled up to the group and introduced myself, and we all started talking. We talked about what we thought the job would entail and how nervous we were.

Someone showed up to let us in. His name was Tim, and he was to be the lead trainer. He welcomed us all into the building. He told everyone to head up to the 3rd floor. Tim and I went up on the elevator. Most of the people had no telecommunications experience. Some did work at a cell phone store. I felt that I had a distinct advantage of seeing I had worked in telecommunications before. We were all given books on what we would learn. The job described to us seemed simple enough. We were to take calls from businesses and handle any questions they had. We would set up any new service that was requested and sell products such as the internet or cell phones. We had to offer any products they didn't already have. The selling part would be new to me. I was confident I could quickly adjust.

I would discover my first major issue with wheelchair accessibility on my break. Usually, how I opened push doors was simple. I would stick my feet straight out and just shove the door open and push until I got through it. As I tried this, the bathroom door barely moved. Most doors have just enough of spring to close the door. The door was so heavy if I took my hands off of my tires, the door would push me back out. Just inside the door was a wall I would also have to navigate.

Not only was I going to have to fight the door, but I had to turn a 90-degree corner. This was not going to be easy. I made it through the door and around the corner. Once I made it around the corner, the door closed behind me. I realized my next issue. At the end of about a 10-foot hallway, there was another tight 90-degree corner. But there was also an enormous trash can in the way. There was barely enough room for a person to get through. I was a bit freaked out. I couldn't go forward because of the trash can. I couldn't back up because of the heavy door shut. I couldn't turn around because I was wedged between the walls.

I had my cell phone on me but didn't have anyone's number. Who was I going to call? I was stuck! I had no clue what to do. Luckily someone from my training class tried to come through the door and found me. He had to climb over me. Then he moved the trash can so I could get through the hallway and around the corner. I rolled into the handicapped stall and started to go to the bathroom. The toilet is required to sit much higher in a handicapped stall in case the disabled person can't bend down. This toilet was much too low.

Once I had finally returned to the training room, I looked at the clock, and I was gone 25 minutes. I just returned to my desk. The union leadership was there to talk to us. They discussed how union dues worked and where the union hall was. They told us if we ever had a problem, we were to go to union leadership as soon as possible. The union leader for our floor was named Joe. They asked if anyone had any questions. I figured now is as good of a time as any. I wondered if I could talk to them privately.

I suggested that we get Tim as well. I wanted him to know the issues as well. I walked them through my problems with the door by demonstrating how I had to open it. I showed them how my chair didn't fit down the hallway. Someone had moved the trash can back. So that was in the way again. I went into the stall and explained the issue with the toilet. Tim said that he would get with his bosses right away and talk to them. Joe said he would get with the other union leaders and see what they could do. He was also going to go to every bathroom in the building.

I was happy with their response. I was anxious that they would not understand. My biggest fear was what would happen if I had to sit down to use the bathroom. If I forced myself to sit down and my knees didn't bend that far, I wouldn't be able to get up. So what was I supposed to do call for help? Both Tim and Joe seemed to understand the issues. We went back into the training room and joined the rest of the class.

A few days later, I met with Joe and the head of the union to discuss the bathroom issues. They had gone through all the bathrooms in the building. Each bathroom was the same way. They said they would still look into things. They planned to have the repairs done by the end of the training. They told me to keep working hard as I could. Tim had already been impressed with my knowledge and how I answered questions.

The only thing I had issues with was putting sales first. Our job was to offer whatever product or service they didn't have. If the customer said no, we had to overcome that objection and close the sale. It is harder than you think. I had always been trained just to do customer service. As training went on, I became more and more comfortable with things. I still knew in the back of my head that I might have an issue with pushing for sales. They trained us never to take no for an answer. We had to sell things that the customer may not need.

Our job was to make them believe that they needed it. There were times that a customer needed what I was selling. Those times were few and far between. Another goal was to get a customer into at least one yearly contract. This would be the first month we would have a monthly scorecard. The scorecard consisted of three parts. Part one was our percentage was of the sales goal. The second part was our call observation score. Each month our manager or, in this case, Tim would listen to a set of 5 calls. The third part was adherence. That counted the amount of time we were taking calls.

Adherence was the amount of time you were on the phone, taking calls during your shift. That number had to be at least 92% in an 8-hour shift left you with roughly 39 minutes to use off the phone. If you needed to leave your desk for any reason, it counted against you. It took me longer to get around than it did everyone else. It became a more significant issue when we moved to the main floor. I figured out that the ramp leading into the office was very steep. I had to be extremely careful not to wheel too hard because my chair would try to flip over backward.

They had already started firing people in the training class. Which made the stress in the training area go sky high. I was doing OK, but I was losing points when it came to overcoming the objection. With a few weeks left of training, some of the class had already moved to their permanent teams. I wrote an email to Tim in asking about the status of modifications we had discussed. A few minutes after sending the email, Tim came up to me carrying a copy of the email. He hadn't heard anything yet.

Several weeks passed, and we had a meeting about the accommodations. They would be putting a button on the outside of the bathroom door. The wall could not be removed, and they refused to change the toilet in the bathroom. They would be getting a seat that fits over the toilet to raise it.

As far as the adherence standards, they told me it was a vital part of the job. They could not change it. They would hold me to the same standards as everyone. I pointed out that it takes me longer to do things such as go to the printer or the bathroom. I told them a provision in the ADA that says they had to. I was advised by the union to let it go. They said if the company wrote me up for it, then they would fix the problem. That seemed backward to me. A few days after my meeting, I passed my final training!

I was excited training was over, but nervous at the same time. My manager Sally came over and hugged me and welcomed me. Sally wanted to talk, so I would know the expectations she had for me. Her expectations were what I expected them to be. I briefly explained some of the issues that I had. My desk was very close to Sally's so I didn't have to move to ask her a question. I was also close to the printer.

I had a meeting with Sally over my December numbers. My sales were well above the goal. My call observations were good. I didn't have good adherence, and they wrote me up. I wasn't happy about it at all. The union said that since the company wrote me up, they would do what they could. I didn't have much faith in anything. Every month I was at or near my sales goals, but my adherence would bring everything down. Each time they wrote me up, I would complain and plead my case. The company said they were working on the issues. The office had a shakeup, and everyone was changing teams. I was now on Lorna's team. I liked Lorna, but she was way different than Sally. She was tough and reminded me of my mom.

Chapter 14

Now that I was working a lot, I missed being a dad. I did the best I could to make time for Lys when and where I could. Lys and I used Saturdays as fun days. We would focus on what we enjoyed doing together. We both love movies. We would go to movies if there were one we wanted to see. Or we would go shopping at the mall. I had never been able to afford new clothes for her, but I could now. She took full advantage of that.

One time I got myself a bit over my head. I had taken a few days off of work. We decided to go to an outlet mall. The mall was dead with hardly anyone there. She wanted to go to Justice because she loves bright colors and glitter. Everything they have seems to fall into those categories. I told Lys she could get a couple of outfits. She did need some summer clothes. She picked out some stuff and wanted to try them on.

Let me set the scene. One female employee was helping Lys try on clothes while the other was picking out more stuff to try on. Before long, there was a huge pile. I started to break out into a cold sweat. I knew this wasn't good. Thankfully I was able to talk her out of a few things, and I had a 40% off coupon. We still ended up with way more than I intended. We didn't go into a Justice for a long time after that. I was too scared to go near one.

Unfortunately for me, Carley also noticed I was making money. She decided to go against our signed agreement and ask me for child support. Our divorce was final for about three years, and she hadn't asked for a dime. Now I was making money, and soon she was coming around with her hand out. As far as I was concerned, we had joint custody. She was responsible for expenses on her week, and I was on mine. I didn't mind paying for school expenses and stuff like that. I just didn't think I should have to help Carley pay her bills. The state did not see my point of view. They ordered me to pay a few hundred dollars a month in child support plus all medical expenses.

Between work and Carley, I needed a distraction. I decided to try dating again. I wasn't looking for anything serious. I wanted someone to have dinner with when Lys was at her mother's. This time I signed up for pay sites. Not long after signing up, the site matched me with Isabelle. We talked for a few weeks. We decided to meet for dinner. Dinner went well, and the conversation moved along amazingly well. She had a son that was around Lys's age, and that made me happy. I preferred to date women with kids.

Isabelle and I were dating for a month. During the weeks I had Lys, we would just talk. Then on weeks I didn't, we would go out to dinner. Things were going along pretty well, and we had talked about meeting the kids. I decided to let her meet Lys. We met at the mall so we could do some shopping and walk around. We went to dinner, and Lys didn't talk much.

On the way home, I asked Lys what she thought. She made sure to let me know her opinion. She said Isabelle seemed nice, but her hair was funny looking. Lys also hated that she kept asking her questions. Lys didn't want me to see her anymore. Lys said if I made her go to dinner with Isabelle again, she wasn't going to talk to her. I was sorry, I asked! I was glad she felt open to telling me her opinion.

We went out to dinner with her again two weeks later. Lys didn't say a word to her the entire time. I was thinking of breaking it off because if Lys didn't like her, it wasn't going to work. I didn't have to make that decision. A few days later, Isabelle called me all upset and informed me she was pregnant by her ex-boyfriend. She felt she had to break up with me and try and figure things out with him. I feel like Lys could sense something about her I couldn't, and she was right.

I wanted to make sure I went to every school event Lys had. I knew they were important to her. The next big school event was a daddy/daughter dance. I wanted the dance to be something special. A few weeks before the dance, we went dress shopping. I didn't want anything to fancy. I did want something beautiful. We went to a few stores, and it became clear that the dress I had in mind and the dress Lys did were two completely different things. I picked out a dress, and I let her pick out a couple.

The dress I picked out was white, and it had some pearls on it. It was beautiful. Lys walked out of the changing room in full attitude. She looked at me and said, "You don't expect me to wear this in public, do you." All I could do was laugh. I knew I wasn't going to win, and this wasn't going to be worth the fight. So I let her pick her dress. The dress was sheer pink with red flowers on it. I got a pink dress shirt and a tie.

One the day of the dance, we went to get her hair done. I explained to the hairdresser Tammy what I wanted, which was kind of a curly up do. Lys's hair was adorable when done. Tammy went the extra mile and did her nails and gave her some pink lip gloss. Tammy asked her if she liked her hair, and she said yes. I could tell by the look on her face that may not be the truth.

When we left the salon, I asked her if she liked her hair. She spun around and glared at me. I knew I was in trouble. Lys pointed to her hair and said she had told me she didn't want poufy hair and look her hair was poufy. She was NOT happy. She chewed me out all the way to the car. I apologized, but that didn't do any good. Things got a little better at the dance when all her friends said they loved her hair.

Unfortunately, work was not going as well for me as fatherhood was. In the months, I complained about all the Americans with Disability Act violations, my sales would drop. In the months I didn't complain my sales were high. I showed Lorna all of the numbers I had. She looked at it and smiled. She said I would think you would learn to keep your mouth shut. I also talked to a person in the union about it. They said if the company decided they wanted to get rid of someone, they could easily do it.

I had a meeting with my union representative Trevon, Lorna, and the department head Karol at Lorna's desk. The meeting got rather heated. They denied that I had ever written the email I had sent to Tim. They were making it clear that I had to get my adherence to an acceptable level, or they may fire me. Karol got so mad at me she stormed off. Trevon pulled me aside and asked me about the email I wrote to Tim. Tim admitted that he had seen it and that he had also given a copy to Karol.

A few days after this, I had another meeting in Karol's office with Trevon. They told me the company would be bringing in an ADA expert to visit with me and look at the facilities. Karol made it clear that they did not believe there were any violations in the building. The expert was supposed to be a non-company employee. The union had agreed that anyone employed by the company might be biased. They told me that they had bought a toilet seat and they would install it in a few days. They were moving my desk to the central aisle of the office. I would also have a new manager named Andy. I wasn't happy with the managerial change. Andy and I did not see eye to eye. I got the feeling from the meeting that it was Andy's job to fire me.

The company was doing all they could to make me quit. I knew it was Andy's job to fire me. I felt like they were mocking me with how they were handling my accommodations. The type of seat they bought just sat on top of the rim of the bowl. I tried to sit on it, and it slid off and fell to the floor. I complained, and the company said that it was the best they were going to do. I complained to Trevon, and he said that there wasn't anything the union could do. I was not happy but felt trapped under the circumstances.

The ADA expert was named Elise, and I was ready for her. I didn't trust the company. I researched the ADA more than I had previously. I was going to ask this expert some questions and make sure she was qualified. Elise came to my desk and looked around. Then she watched as I wheeled through the office then down the ramp. I started quizzing her carefully with a few questions. Most of which she seemed to ignore.

After the 4th question, she asked why I kept asking her questions about the ADA. She admitted she did not know the ADA. She was a business ergonomics expert. She was an expert on sitting at your desk correctly and that sort of thing. When I mentioned that the company had told me she was an ADA expert, she laughed and said no. I was irate because they lied to me. As soon as Elise left, I went and had a chat with Trevon. I told him what Elise had said to me about not knowing anything about the ADA. Trevon immediately went in to talk to Karol because they lied to him as well.

The new plan was to bring in an expert from a local hospital. Karol assured me that he was an expert. Karol also promised that whatever the expert found was in violation would be fixed. They wanted me to agree if the expert found no violations, I would stop complaining. I agreed as long as it was a third party expert with no ties to the company. We both decided that the terms were acceptable. Karol introduced me to Robert and his assistant Trish. Robert was knowledgeable about the ADA and its requirements. He also assured me that he would give an honest evaluation of the building.

Robert and I went through the entire building. We went from the parking lot up to the office and through the bathroom facilities. I just wanted an opportunity to work on an even playing field. Robert and Trish measured the ramp and told me that it was 2 feet shorter than regulation. He also said that if I had a motorized chair, the incline was so steep it would ruin the motor. Robert advised me that the bathroom was unusable and dangerous. He also found many other violations, including the front door. I spent all morning with Robert. He said he would give his report to the company in a few days. After Robert left, I had a meeting with Trevon and Karol to make sure I found Robert acceptable. I said I did and was very pleased although I wanted to see the report.

Several weeks later, I was called into Karol's office because Robert's report was in. Robert's report was only two pages, but it went through several violations and fixes. Karol said she was shocked by all the violations. She also said that she couldn't believe that the ramp leading to the office was illegal. They sent a copy to the corporate office and that the repairs would begin very soon.

As part of the recommended changes by Robert, the company decided to build a handicapped bathroom. It took them about a year to build it. Sadly it wasn't built up to code. They used a regular toilet in it and not a disabled one. When I pointed this out, they told me that's the only one they had. I had to just deal with it. I was made aware that they were re-measuring the ramp. I asked who and what their qualifications were. The men measuring the ramp worked for the company. I could see them measuring the ramp from my desk. It was my break time, so I went to get a closer look.

I went down the ramp and pretended to be on my cell phone while watching them. The men stopped what they were doing and stood in front of the ramp. They told me I was not allowed to see what they were doing. They would not continue until I was back at work. A few days later, Karol advised me the ramp had been re-measured and was legal. They said it was the railing leading up the ramp that was illegal. I had been there when Robert measured the ramp. I know damn well he didn't even touch the railing, let alone measure it.

One good thing happened around this time. I got a new manager named Norma. Norma and I always had a great relationship before she became a manager. I knew she respected the work I did for the customers. I hoped she wouldn't be as underhanded as Andy was. Norma and I had a meeting at her desk. She asked me to lay out all my issues on the table. All she asked was that maybe I tone it down I bit. I agreed that I would work hard for her.

Things with Norma went very smoothly. Then I was passed over for a promotion because my adherence was too low. I went to Norma, and we had a long talk about it. I expressed my frustration about the adherence policy and reminded her that I had been complaining about it since I started. Norma said she would have to talk to Karol, and she would get back to me.

A few days later, I was in a meeting with Norma, Karol, and two union representatives Chuck and Marie. The meeting was in regards to the adherence policy. From the time the meeting started, Karol was very agitated. She said that it was a vital metric to the job, and I was lucky I hadn't been written up more for it. I started pointing out the flaws with it. I timed myself, and it took me 3 minutes to go to the printer. I asked Chuck and Marie how long it took them. They both said less than a minute. I pointed out that it took me about 15 minutes or more to use the bathroom. Chuck said it took him about 4 minutes, and Marie said around 5. Karen started getting all red in the face and yelling at me. I refused to back down! I have been fighting with them for years, and I have had enough!

I was determined to finish it right here and right now. I also brought up that if it weren't for the adherence trouble, I would have been a service leader. Karol said that the service leader had to move around the office from desk to desk. She did not think I could do that fast enough. I would never be allowed to be a service leader. I then asked her if she can recognize the fact, then why not the same things in regards to adherence.

Instead of answering my question, she told me to get out of her office. I was not going to leave until we had settled the issues. She grabbed Norma by the arm and stormed off. When they left, Chuck and Marie just looked at me, stunned. About five minutes later, Norma and Karol returned. Karol started yelling again, but she said she had a deal for me.

Karol said that she would waive my adherence portion of my scorecard and give me the full points for it. Then when the building was ADA compliant, I was to be held by the same standard as everyone. I agreed to the deal because that building was never going to be 100% compliant. Even the handicapped bathroom they built wasn't compliant. She demanded that Chuck and Marie get me out of her office. A few months after our meeting, Karol announced she was transferring, and we would have a new director named Jeanette.

Chapter 15

With all the stress from work, I decided Lys, and I would take a vacation. The place I most wanted to go to was Disney. I wasn't sure if we could handle a week at Disney. I was worried about how we would get to the parks and from the airport to the hotel. I called Disney and asked them all my questions. They have the Disney Magical Express from the airport to my hotel. I wouldn't even have to get our bags from the baggage claim. They would send us tags to put on our bags. The bags would go straight from the plane to our room. The hotels have busses with wheelchair access to every park Disney has, including their Downtown Disney shopping district. I decided to book the trip.

Before I knew it, we were packing to get ready to leave. I had flown before, but Lys never had, so she was nervous. Going through airport security in a wheelchair is a trick. They pull people in wheelchairs to the side. They swab the chair and my shoes and on and on. The flight attendant picked up on Lys being nervous and started talking to her. She took her to meet the pilot and showed her the cockpit. When Lys had to go to the bathroom, the flight attendant helped her. She guarded the door and made sure Lys got back to her seat.

Once we landed and were off the plane, they had a porter escort us to the Magical Express. Disney assured us our luggage would be at our room later. We got to the hotel, and we had to wait for about an hour before our room would be ready. Lys wanted to go swimming in the pool. She wanted to enjoy the few days of warm weather, seeing it was winter back in Michigan.

Our first day would be at Hollywood Studios. We got up and had breakfast because there is no better way to start a day at Disney than with a Mickey waffle. We loved Hollywood studious! We had fun on all the rides and at all the shows. There was so much to do. We did end up going on the Toy

Story ride several times. We loved it so much. They had a particular car they just rolled me into while I stayed in my chair.

The next day we were headed to Epcot. I also had scheduled a special breakfast. Lys loves Stitch, so I had to make sure we made Breakfast with Stitch. Lys usually isn't a kid who loves characters in big outfits. But at Disney, she was in love with them. Especially when Stitch came around, she loved it and kept hugging him. I loved the look on her face. It made the cost of the trip worth every penny. I think she would have been perfectly fine following Stitch around all day long.

We rode the monorail back to Epcot and got off and entered the park. There is so much to do at Epcot, especially in the countries. One of the things we did was a 4D movie experience called Honey I Shrunk the Audience. The experience is just like the movie Honey I shrunk the Kids. We got in, and we soon noticed we were seated next to a large group. They must have been on a day trip with a bunch of aides. The basic premise is much like the movie. Rick Moranis accidentally shrinks the audience, and then the audience goes through a few experiences. The whole thing is pretty cool.

What makes it different for this story is the group we are sitting in the middle of. I guess they couldn't process the fact that it's not real. They started freaking out, thinking they have been shrunk and are about to be stepped on. So the aides tried to get them out of there. But they think I am part of their group because I am sitting in the middle of them. Lys was yelling at them to leave her daddy alone!

Next, we were going to the Animal Kingdom Park, which is the smallest of the parks. I will admit Animal Kingdom is my least favorite of the Disney Parks. I don't like how Disney designed it. It's the least wheelchair-friendly of the parks. When they made it, they wanted it to have a more rustic look. The streets and walkways are very rough and bumpy. Which is hard on someone in a wheelchair, and it's hilly. We went straight to the safari, and that was cool. Then we did sit for a few of the animal shows. They have a short version of The Lion King Broadway show. I would love to see the full show someday. We had seen everything we wanted to in just a few hours, and we left. Lys wanted to go to Downtown Disney for some shopping.

One thing I wanted Lys to do was to get made up like a princess. They had a salon called the Bippity Boppity Boutique, and it was adorable. They do the girls' hair and a little makeup to look like a princess. I had begged Lys to do it. She kept saying she wasn't a girly girl. One of the boutique locations was in a store in Downtown Disney. We were in the store looking around. She picked up this painting and art kit she wanted. I told her no because it was expensive. She must have wanted it because she said if I bought it for her, she would let them make her a princess.

I checked with the boutique, and they had an open appointment. I thought we were just doing hair and makeup, but Lys said she wanted the full princess outfit. They said they would be more than happy to do that for her. She chose princess Jasmine because she said Jasmine is the only princess that wears pants. For as much as she claims not to be a girly girl, she loved the makeover. She started to get into it. Before I knew it, I had Princess Lys. The workers at Disney can tell once a girl has had the princess makeover. The look stays for several days. The rest of the trip, they called her princess, and some would even curtsy to her. It was so cute!

Our last day, we were at the Magic Kingdom. We would also be going to Mickey's Merry Christmas Party. The party is another ticket you have to buy. There are a limited number of tickets. They also have special stage performances, a special parade, and a special fireworks display. As the party approached, they made several announcements warning people. If you didn't have a wristband for the party would have to leave. We made sure to get our wristbands early. The lines to the rides are also much shorter.

Disney had characters out in special Christmas outfits. Lys had to wait in line for a picture with Holiday Stitch. Then later, we found him again dressed up as Santa Stitch. I had to laugh because she wouldn't wait in a line longer than 20 minutes for a ride. However, she would wait in a massive line for Stitch. Disney has select roped off areas, especially for people in wheelchairs for the parade. Everything was so festive and just over the top. I think the week allowed Lys and I to grow closer. This week was only the two of us. After the final holiday fireworks, we headed to the bus while we sang Christmas carols. We had a fantastic night. There are not many places where being disabled isn't an issue. Disney is so accessible and amazing!

When I got back from vacation, I was moved to a new manager Jake. He questioned my adherence and said he knew of the deal I had with Karol. He also let me know that part of his monthly bonus had to do with team adherence. He wanted me to try and get it better. He was willing to help me where ever he could. Another problem happening now was that people were using the handicapped bathroom when they didn't need to. So many times, I had to wait 10 minutes or more to get into the bathroom, but Jeanette said she couldn't stop people from using it.

A few months after, I was at Jake's desk, going over my scorecard. I was in for a shock. Jake told me the company was not going to stick within the deal I made with Karol. They were going to write me up. They screwed me over. I went over to both Marie and Chuck, and they both said that they couldn't do it because we had a deal. Both Jeanette and Jake held their ground, and the union let it slide. Jake did sit down with me. We tried to come up with a plan to get my adherence to an acceptable level. Jake came up with health sheets.

I would write down every time I was away from my desk. I would turn it in and get the time waived when we started doing that my adherence was at an acceptable level. This went on for a few weeks. Then they came to me and said the only thing that was allowed to go on the sheets were bathroom breaks. I asked for the hundredth time to have a printer put at my desk. They said they couldn't do that. Every time I thought we were finally getting somewhere, they would kick me back a step. I was beyond frustrated!

Chapter 16

Work may have been a mess, but things with Lys were good. Until I picked her up from Carley's, and she seemed upset. I asked her why she was upset. Lys explained that her mother was gone all the time. Lys said that she wouldn't see her mother much. She said her mother would leave not long after she got home from school and wouldn't come home till she was already asleep. To top it off, Carley came over to pick Lys up at the end of the week. Lys wasn't ready yet. Carley sat on my couch and made some phone calls. She called a friend and made sure of their plans to go out that night. Carley was picking Lys up just to drop her off and go to the bar. I demanded to keep Lys if she was going to be out all night. She refused to do it, and she grabbed Lys and took her.

I did the only thing I could do. I called Child Protective Services in the morning and made a report. I told them everything that Lys had said. They told me that they would pass it on to a worker. They advised me to call back in twenty-four hours. I called the next day, and they opened a case. I had a phone interview. She said she would go out to their house and the kid's school. I knew soon after she went to their house. Carley called me when I was at work. She was irate that I had called on her.

I admitted I did it, and I didn't care. Carley really couldn't do a damn thing about it. She tried to file a charge on me saying that I couldn't take care of Lys. That got dismissed rather quickly. I may have worked a lot, but I made sure Lys was more than taken care of. Carley refused even to call the worker back. When she went to the house, they wouldn't answer the door. Carley knew they would want to talk to the kids. She had time to coach the kids on what to say and what not to say. I think had the worker gone to the school first and talked to the kids right away; things would have turned out better.

After the worker talked to the kids, she called me. She said they wouldn't speak to her. She had no doubt what I was saying was true. The worker needed Lys to admit it. When she finally was able to talk to Carley, she was very argumentative and blamed me for being an angry ex. Another issue I had is the worker didn't see a problem with Carley leaving the kids home alone because Noah was twelve. They said he was old enough. I pointed out that Noah had Asperger's Autism. They said that had no bearing on anything. This was so frustrating.

Now that I knew the state wouldn't help me. I had to take as many steps as I could to make sure that Lys was safe. I had met their neighbor at a couple of the kid's birthday parties and befriended her. I made sure she had my number and my mom's. She did tell me that the kids did come over to play with her grandson. I told Lys to go there if she needed to.

The neighbor assured me she would always be there for them. There was also a small corner store a block away that the kids could walk to. I gave Lys money just in case they needed food, and the neighbor wasn't home. I also took the step to get Lys a cell phone. The phone wasn't much. It was a pink flip phone. I programmed all the numbers she would need into it. She could text, so if I was at work, she could text me. I showed her how to use it, and she was thrilled.

This way, I could call her, or she could contact me if she needed to. I wasn't spoiling her. I just wanted her to be safe. The only thing that happened was Carley let Noah borrow it once. He answered when I called to talk to Lys. I had to get a court order barring Carley or anyone in her home from touching Lys's phone. I paid the bill so Carley couldn't take it from her. She couldn't use it, and Carley couldn't even tell Lys to let anyone else use it.

I hated going that extra step, but I had to. I had to be one step ahead as much as possible. I also went to school and talked to anyone and everyone I could. I met with the principal, her teachers, and the school counselor. I informed them about what was going on. They promised to keep an eye on her. I made sure she had extra money on her lunch account. On the days Lys didn't get breakfast, she knew to tell someone, and they would take care of her. I hated relying on all these other people, but I was working a lot. I should have been able to rely on Carley to do these things. She was more worried about her Life and not Lys's.

The hardest part about being a single dad and dealing with Carley's crap is I didn't take much time for myself. Between working and taking care of Lys, that's is all I seemed to do. You get to a point where you forget to take time for yourself. With what little free time I had, I enjoyed playing cards online. This was my way of social interaction without having to leave my house. One day in the online game room, I met Raquel. She was somewhat crazy in a wild way. I will admit I kind of liked that.

She lived near Toledo, which was only a few hours away. I had no intention of ever meeting her. We talked online. Then we started talking on the phone. Raquel even sent me some pictures. They were of her in a full leather dominatrix outfit. I am not into that kind of thing, but at the same time, I did like the pictures. We had talked for a few months, and she asked me if I would come to visit her. I wasn't sure that was a good idea. I didn't know her at all. Before I answered her, I looked her up everywhere I could. I ran her home number through the system at work and got her last name. Then I googled her and did all the research I could. You just can never be too careful.

After thinking it over, I decided to meet Raquel. The plan was to drive down on a Saturday and have dinner and stay the night. Then drive back home on Sunday. The entire way down, I kept thinking I was insane. I had told friends where I was going and what the plan was. I didn't dare tell my family. I made it down there safe. The one thing she did that bothered me was Raquel smoked. Other than that we had a great dinner and I had booked a room in a nice hotel.

Had I not been in a wheelchair, I would have just gone to her place. I couldn't do that, so I did the next best option. Instead of going to a movie, we cuddled and watched a movie on in the room. We did fool around some. I wasn't comfortable enough to go further. I had never had a one night stand, and I wasn't about to have one now. She wanted more and tried several times to go further, but something kept telling me not to. I did enjoy the evening. The next morning we talked about meeting up again.

We continued to talk over the next few weeks. There was an odd twist in some of the conversations. Raquel would bring up parenthood from time to time. Then pay me compliments on what a great father I was. Before I had gone to see her, we never talked like that. I won't say what we talked about before. Let's just say our talks did get very risqué from time to time. Now they had switched to a more family-oriented nature. I found it a bit odd. I just wasn't sure why that had happened. Raquel had made it clear she wanted to see me again. I knew she wasn't trying to scare me off or get rid of me.

A month after I had been down for a visit, she told me that she had found out she was pregnant by her ex-boyfriend. I didn't know what to do. Seriously what are the odds this could happen to me twice? We both decided just to be friends. She did send me pictures of her son several months later. I wonder had we done more if she would have tried to pin the kid on me. She did comment many times on how great of a dad I was and how I made good money. I will never know for sure, but it did make me think.

Just as things with Raquel had ended, Life reminded again why I needed to stay focused on Lys. Her teacher said that she couldn't stay focused in class. She would get distracted by the smallest of things. The more noise in class, the worse it would get. I did start to blame her for it. I told her she just needed to try harder. In my mind, if she wanted to focus in school, she would. She wasn't flunking. She was closer to failing than she needed to be. I knew she was smarter than what she was showing. At home, she would breeze through schoolwork. When she would go to school and take tests, she would just lose her train of thought. I set out to have her tested.

I didn't tell Carley a thing. I didn't want her to fight me on it. I had all the tests done, and I talked to several doctors. They suggested I put her on a pill called Focalin. All she had to do was take one every morning before school. Once she started taking the pills, her grades went way up. She went from near failing to being an honor roll student. The change was dramatic.

The only problem was that with our custody arrangement, I only had Lys every other week. I still didn't think Carley would give her the pill. My mom would drive into the school every morning and make sure she took it. This went on for months until Lys let it slip to Carley. Carley chewed me out in a very one-sided fight. Granted, she had a point, but I still believed in my decision at the time.

With Lys doing so well in school, I decided to try dating again. I had met someone on EHarmony named Deena. She worked for the newsroom of a local TV station. I liked her because she was just different than most of the girls I had ever dated. She was very much a free spirit and an artsy person. She even played roller derby in her spare time. She was about eight years younger than me. I didn't have an issue with it; she sure did. She kept bringing it up all the time.

She didn't mind the fact that I was in a wheelchair because her mom had been in one when she was growing up. Our first date was a simple dinner and a movie. It was one of the best first dates I had ever had. We talked and talked and just enjoyed each other's company. I invited her back to my apartment. We watched another movie and just talked and cuddled on the couch. It was a perfect date that lasted until about 4 am. She said she had to go because she didn't want to go too far too fast. While I did agree with her, I will admit I was disappointed at the same time.

Deena and I talked every day for hours. She would bring over the strangest movies. I watched several with her that were foreign movies with subtitles. I loved spending time with her because I never knew what to expect but in the right way. One of the best dates we went and saw an African ballet. I didn't think I would like it, but it was terrific. I thought maybe Deena was the one.

We had a problem. Deena wanted nothing to do with Lys. She only came over a couple of times when Lys was home. Deena made sure Lys was asleep before she came over. One time that hurt the most was she called from work. We were talking, and she wanted to come over. Instead of asking if Lys was home, she asked if I was free or if I had other responsibilities. That hurt and broke my heart. As much as I liked Deena, I knew I couldn't date her anymore. I couldn't let anyone, no matter how much I loved them, come between Lys and me. So once she said that I started distancing myself. I didn't bother fighting over it because it wasn't worth it. We had a long talk, and I told her we should stop seeing each other. I was heartbroken, but I know I made the right decision.

Chapter 17

I didn't wait long before jumping back into the dating game. I was still playing in the card room online, where I met Raquel. I was talking to a woman in the room named Olivia. I had been talking to Olivia for months online. We realized that we lived 15 minutes from each other. She had just separated from her husband. She had a son named Eric that was a few years younger than Lys. We were soon talking on the phone every day. Olivia was fiery and kind of a bitch. She didn't seem to be interested in meeting at first. I was starting too really like her, but I didn't push things. I valued her friendship. The apartment was lonely when Lys wasn't here, and I needed the attention.

Finally, after a few months, we agreed to meet for dinner. I was excited. Then just a few hours before I was to meet Olivia, she sent me an email. She had decided to give her marriage another try. She thought it best if we no longer talked so she could concentrate on her marriage. I felt heartbroken! I had even bought her flowers on the way home from work. I didn't know what to do. I didn't call her because she asked me not to. I did email her back and told her I understood her wishes, but I was still upset.

I didn't have long to wait for Olivia to contact me. She called me a few days later after her, and her husband fought. Every time she fought with him, she called me. Several times I was woken up around 3 am with her upset on the phone. I always talked to her, no matter what. Olivia admitted to me that she knew her marriage was over. Her husband had been cheating on her. Olivia knew what she had to do for her and Eric. She just needed the strength to do it. I understood this because I had been through the same thing when I was with Carley. I walked her through the process and what she would need to do. I even helped her pick an attorney.

We were getting closer than ever. We finally met for dinner. As it turns out, Olivia's favorite restaurant was the same one I took Lys to for kid's nights. She was pretty. The one thing I noticed right away was she was very loud. When she talked, everyone could hear her. Her personality was huge. When she walked into a room, everyone knew it. You could feel her presence. Her personality was bigger than life. Olivia also was a huge sports fan, especially football. She loved the Lions and the Wolverines as much as I did. I was already falling in love. Nothing is sexier than a woman who loves football.

The dinner and drinks went great. We agreed to do it again real soon. We even talked when we got home. We had dinner a few more times, always at the same spot. Her custody arraignment was the same as mine, so it was easy to meet up. Soon we decided to get together with the kids and see how that went. To keep things fun and easy, I suggested we meet up for bowling. That way, the kids could get to know each other while they were playing. The kids got along excellent, and it wasn't long before they were laughing and teasing each other. They acted like they had known each other for years and not just minutes. Seeing bowling went so well we then decided to go to dinner. The kids demanded to sit next to each other, and they played games together and talked and laughed.

Olivia and I were delighted with how things were going. Olivia said Eric usually took a long time to warm up to people, but he loved us right away. He was very high strung and very energetic. He did take some getting used to. Lys was a quiet kid who could keep herself entertained. Eric always wanted someone to be entertaining him. Olivia had to travel for work on occasion. When she needed a sitter for Eric, I would do it. Many times he stayed with us while Olivia was out of town. Lys loved having him there, and they never had any issues. Having Eric around really filled the hole I had in my heart from losing Noah.

I don't want it to seem like Olivia, and I didn't have our issues because we did. She seemed to be very unsure about our relationship at times. I chalked some of it up to her going through a divorce. I remembered how I was with Holly not long after my divorce. I tried not to push things with her. She had a nasty habit of going off on me for no reason, especially if she had been drinking. She would call me up and start a fight with me over nothing. Then she would call a few days later and pull me back in.

The worst times were on Thursdays. She was in a bowling league on Thursdays and would drink too much. Then after bowling, she would call me late. She would always start a fight. She would call me Friday morning and apologize. To this day, I have no idea why I would answer the phone when she called. I cared about her, and I would have done anything for her. Olivia started talking about moving in together. I was all for the idea. She said before we could do it, she would have to sell her condo. Then we could start looking for a place together. We had hoped that we could find a wheelchair, accessible house. We checked into options on getting a house-made wheelchair accessible.

Olivia got a realtor for her condo and started getting it ready to sell. One problem she had was she had a cat named Tubbers. Her realtor suggested that she find somewhere else for the cat. Lys had always wanted a pet, so I said we would take Tubbers. The only problem I had then was my apartment was supposed to be a pet-free building. I did some research and found out that under the Americans with Disabilities act you could get any animal declared an emotional support animal. So now we had Tubbers, the support cat.

As I look back now, there were a lot of warning signs about Olivia. I just didn't want to see them. She either had the worst luck of any human alive, or she lied to me a ton. She was a major drama queen! She seemed to love chaos and loved just to cause emotional turmoil. Olivia had Multiple Sclerosis, and those symptoms were similar to the symptoms that I have. If I had a day, I wasn't feeling well; then, she would instantly feel worse. If something happened to me or someone she knew, then something would happen to her but worse.

Now that I look back at things, it was a lot like those catfish stories you hear about today. Where the person has one major medical issue after another, or they have car accidents one after another. That was Olivia, without a doubt. Once she told me she had cervical cancer. She wasn't sure what she was going to do. She said she needed major surgery and faced a long recovery time. We talked about her moving in with me because all of the handicapped adaptations were perfect for someone having major surgery. Then a few weeks later, she said her doctor misdiagnosed her.

Olivia lost her job a few weeks after she put her condo on the market. It was a few months before she found another job, which put a significant strain on her finances. Her new job was a much longer drive, and with her finances a mess, she needed money for gas. Being the guy that I am, I offered to help. I gave her an ATM card of mine and told her the PIN. I wasn't too worried about it because I had a small limit set on it. We talked, and she promised not to overdo it.

Around this time, work wanted me to take some night classes. They said it would be good for me and could lead to a promotion. The classes did mean that I would have some extremely long days. I would be working 8-5 every day, then going to class from 6-10, which was rough. My entire day would be from 7 am when I left, and I wouldn't get home till 11 pm, and I would do this for two months.

All I was doing was working and going to class. I was so exhausted. I knew I had to push through it. Near the end of my classes, I went to get gas, and it declined my card. I knew I should have had close to seven thousand in my account. I usually knew how much was in there. Between work and my classes, I hadn't looked at my account in weeks. When I went online and looked at my account, I was stunned. All my money was gone. I didn't even know what to do.

My first problem was I needed gas to get home, and I had no money. I had to borrow money from a friend to get home. That was as humiliating as it gets. I called Olivia to see what in the hell she had done. She claimed she had no clue what I was talking about. She told me how much she had taken out with the ATM and said she didn't take thousands.

I got home and went through every transaction for the last two months. I slowly pieced things together. Somehow and I am still not sure how Olivia got my check card number. She hadn't used the ATM card much, but she sure as hell used my check card number. I have never been so upset in my life. Even when Carley cheated on me, it wasn't this bad. I didn't even know where to start. I had no clue how I would get to work because I had no money for gas. I had no clue how I would eat. I hadn't bought groceries for a while. I saw charges ranging from gambling websites to car payments and her other bills.

She had even charged a subscription to EHarmony to my check card. I called Olivia again, and we had a huge fight; she was still claiming she didn't do it.

I had no choice but to take the day off of work. The next day I went to my bank for help. By the time I got to the bank, bills had tried to clear, and I was in a huge mess. Thankfully the person I was working with at the bank was amazing. I was freaking out and in tears. My life was a mess, and I was begging for help. The bank waived all the bonce check fees. They could tell something strange had happened. Then they arraigned a small loan for me to cover the bills I had written and secured me a credit card I could use.

My bank even went so far as to go through the transaction numbers. They wanted to see the name on the accounts. And it was Olivia's on all of them. They said they would try and get some of it back. They were not sure how that would go. I filed charges with the bank and with the police. Sadly I only got a few hundred returned. She knew I had Lys to take care of, and she didn't give a shit. I ended up with enormous anxiety and depression issues. Olivia did try and get her cat back. I told her I would give her the cat back when I get my money back. I still have the cat!

Even though my finances were a mess, we needed another vacation. We decided to do a four day Disney cruise. Lys had already looked up all there was to do on the ship. I started looking at excursions we could do on the islands. We would be spending one day in the Bahamas and one day on Disney's private island. Disney had a list of things you could do that was a little extra at both locations.

The problem was they didn't have any excursions for people with disabilities. There were a few that I could have done, but the transportation to the locations was by bus. They did not have any busses with lifts. I would have to be able to get on and off the bus myself. I knew I couldn't do that. They had a bunch of cool things listed for the private island. Such as feeding stingrays. I knew Lys would have loved to do, but everything said it involved stairs. I was shocked because Disney always seemed to wheelchair friendly. I was sure the cruise would be the same way. I was learning the hard way that it wasn't.

I called Disney to see if they had anything to help or any excursions not listed. The phone call with Disney went about as bad as it could have. They told me there was nothing they can do. Disney said the private island was in international waters and therefore was not bound by American laws. And our days in the Bahamas were outside of America. There are not any laws such as the American with Disabilities Act in the Bahamas. I didn't give up and started emailing my way up the chain of Disney. I had hope that I could get some kind of change or help. That, however, never happened. This was the first time in my dealings with Disney, where I was disappointed. I thought about canceling the cruise at one point. I talked it over with Lys, and we decided to go ahead with the trip.

When we got to the ship, it was incredible! Everything was Disney, and we loved it! We went to the room and investigated that. I was worried about the bathroom. I knew because it was a ship that everything would be smaller. I was afraid I would have issues getting into the bathroom. While it was small, Disney designed it perfectly. A lot of things were moveable to maximize space. Whoever designed it did a great job. Getting around the ship was a bit complicated. They had huge metal ledges about 6 inches high that made getting over them hard. There were a few marked with handicapped signs that were not as high. The workers were always there to try and help. Luckily I was in a manual chair because I don't think you could get a power chair over them.

There was a lot to do on the ship, and we were having a blast. Lys made a couple of friends. She would make plans to meet up and play basketball or many other things they had to do. They also had clubs for the kids. There was a lot to do for adults as well. The most amazing part was all the food on the cruise was paid for. It was four days of all you can eat, and we did just that. The only extra thing was alcohol. On the first night on the ship, there was a massive party with a bunch of characters, especially Stitch.

There were three main dining rooms. Each night we had dinner in a different one. My favorite dining room was the animation one. As we started dinner, everything on the walls was black and white. As dinner progressed, more and more color would show up. By the end of dinner, everything was full color. It was awesome. Even the uniforms of the wait staff would change. Each dining room had its unique dishes. There were also a few things that were on every menu. I tried to eat some random stuff just to sample different food. The great thing about our waiter was if you couldn't decide on an appetizer, he would bring you two. Torn on what dessert you want here have two and at no additional charge. The food was all delicious.

They also had a movie theater that showed recently released Disney and Pixar movies. One thing we did that we both loved was every night we played bingo. This was as close to gambling that they had. You could win some serious money and other prizes. We did almost break even every night.

The night before we were on the private island, we did win a free excursion. But because it was not wheelchair friendly, we couldn't take it. We would have been able to take a bike trip around the island and pet stingrays. I know Lys would have loved it. We ended up with a Disney T-shirt instead, which was 2nd place in the drawing. I was pissed about it, but there was no point in making a big scene. I did my best to blow it off.

The day in the Bahamas was very uneventful. When we got up in the morning, the boat was already docked at the port. We went and had breakfast, and then we left the ship. The port was in a shopping district. We went through some of the shops and looked around for a while. We had one incident that kind of left a bad taste in our mouths. We were in the shopping district in what looked like a flea market. There were these ladies with a bunch of pretty necklaces. Lys looked at them but decided not to get one. As we were walking away, the lady said she would give one to Lys for free. I said, are you sure and she said yes. So Lys said thank you and picked out a blue coral one. Just as we were about to walk away, the lady stepped in front of us and demanded a donation.

I had two choices. I could just pay for the necklace seeing it was only $7 and get the hell out of there, or I could make a bigger deal about the apparent shakedown. Lys was ready to argue, but I stopped her. I just paid the lady the $7. Lys was still protesting as we left. I explained to her that we were now in a foreign country, and they did things differently there. But it did leave me with a very uneasy feeling. After that, we walked around a bit then had lunch at a restaurant on the water. I still wish we had been able to go to the water park or some of the other cool stuff. I didn't even see any regular taxis I may have been able to make work. All I saw were small busses or full-size vans. Lys then said what I was thinking. She said the ship was more fun. So we just went back to the boat and enjoyed the activities they had.

The next day we went to the private island called Castaway Key. They had things I would have done, but they had no wheelchair access. Lys was too young to do them by herself. Lys was a bit disappointed, but she was happy to spend the day at the beach. They did tell me they had beach wheelchairs that I was free to use. So we planned on doing that.

We found the beach wheelchairs and quickly figured out they were not easy to get into. I almost fell when someone saw me struggling and threw me into it. Then it was too big and bulky for Lys to push. They helped and kind of parked me under a tree. I had a waiter that checked on me and brought me food and drinks. Lys played in the sand and water with one of her friends. While the island wasn't as much fun as I would have liked, it still was pretty cool. They had the real Black Pearl from the movie Pirates of the Caribbean near the beach. People could go and look at it. I hated not being able to move, but Lys had fun, and that is all that mattered.

That night was our last on the ship, and we played bingo. Then walked around the ship and enjoyed the fresh sea air. We had to have our bags outside our rooms that night so they could send them through customs. With everyone's bags in the hallways, it made getting around a bit complicated. The hallways were small, to begin with. There were times Lys just plowed forward and ran stuff over. The next morning we got dressed and had one last breakfast on the ship. It felt funny to be on solid ground again. We could still feel the ship move a few days after the cruise.

We did enjoy the cruise; it was a lot of fun. I would admit it could have been better, especially if Disney had wheelchair accessible things to do on their island and in the Bahamas. I was disappointed at times for sure. The good times outweighed the bad. I understand that Disney wasn't under any legal obligation to do anything as far as accessibility. That doesn't mean they shouldn't have.

That comes down to the issues I have with the world. People and businesses tend to the bare minimum as far as making things accessible. They know most of the time they will never get called out for it. I wish we would have a time where businesses do what is right. Not because they have to but because they want to. Would I recommend a Disney cruise for someone in a wheelchair? Yes, I actually would. They need to understand where the struggles will be and what the limitations are.

Chapter 18

When I returned to work after vacation, I had to get used to a new boss Sheryl. Sheryl cleared it with Jeanette so that I could write any time I needed on my health sheets. My overall scorecard was one of the highest in the office. However, I now had a new issue to worry about. I had been in a lot of pain, and I went to the doctor. They discovered a cyst on my tailbone. The cyst was growing, and it was putting pressure on nerves causing significant pain. I was taking pain pills like candy to get through the day. After I had my surgery, my doctor said he couldn't give me a recovery time. He advised me to stay out of my wheelchair as much as possible. Healing was slow and painful.

I was on short term disability. My doctor was sending notes to the company every two weeks, so they knew how the healing was going. The company said that according to their guidelines, I was only allowed to be off for 12 weeks. I talked to my doctors, and they said I could go back. I still had to see them for bandage changes and cleaning. I would need to go to the doctor 2-3 times a week while working.

On my first day back, I had a meeting with Sheryl. I discussed with her that I would need to still go to the doctor. She said that she would talk to Jeanette. Sheryl came to speak to me. The company would not allow me to go to the doctor. I called my short term disability caseworker. She said that if my doctor had filled out the paperwork outlining what days I needed to go to the doctor, they would have allowed it. I was already back at work, so my case was closed.

I called my doctor's office to see what they had to say. My doctor told me they mentioned to the caseworker that I needed bandage changes. My caseworker told the doctor I had to work it out with my supervisor. They were furious that the company was now refusing to allow it. I went to my union. Weeks went by, and no word from the union. The only way I could get through the day was pain pills. I felt blitzed out of my mind, thanks to the pills. My numbers started to slip.

Sheryl suggested that I think about filing for permanent disability. With the amount of pain I was in, I did think about it. Things went on like this for months. I would ask Sheryl for time to go to the doctor, and she would deny it. I would beg the union for help. They would tell me they were working on it. I talked with Sheryl and asked her what the process was for medical retirement. Once I seemed open to the idea, it was a weekly conversation.

We were working a lot of overtime. The pain was horrible. I was downing a lot of pills just trying to survive. I woke up one day and tried to sit in my chair and I couldn't. The pain was so bad I couldn't do it. I called into work and went to the doctor. They told me that I had a nasty infection. They said if I even tried to work, it would get worse. A month passed, and I was feeling a million times better. I called Sheryl and mentioned coming back to work. She was afraid if I did that, they would fire me. She advised me to go on permanent medical leave.

I ran the money, and I would be able to make it work financially. I wouldn't have much extra money each month. I knew we would have all the bills paid. I did involve Lys in the decision. I wanted her to know what was going on and the changes we would be making. I told her that we would be fine, but we wouldn't be going shopping unless we needed something. I said we would still do some stuff, but we would have to watch the money we were spending. She looked right at me and hugged me. She said she didn't care about any of that. All she wanted was her daddy. As she did that I retired and it was the best decision.

Chapter 19

Just as life was going well for Lys and me, we got some devastating news. Carley came to pick Lys up and go to her house. Later I got a call from Lys saying Kyle had just died. I was so shocked. I thought I didn't hear her right. I made her repeat it. Lys told me Kyle had a heart attack and died. I talked to Carley to see how she was. I was worried about her. Carley said she was OK just in shock.

Kyle had no life insurance or health insurance. This was going to be a massive mess for her. Another problem was Kyle was the breadwinner of the house. I talked to Carley; she had enough money for about six months' worth of bills. She wasn't sure what she would do after that. She filled me in on the funeral details. I decided I would go to support her and be there for Lys. I felt like I still had to be there, so Carley knew I cared.

When I got Lys back home, I sat her down for a long talk. I needed information so I could better understand what happened. Lys said Kyle started not feeling well when she got there. He was lying in the bathroom on the floor. Carley wanted to call an ambulance, but Kyle said no. Carley was with him in the bathroom, and suddenly he lost consciousness. Carley called 911.

When the paramedics got there, Lys went into vivid detail as they tried to revive him. She saw things no child should see. They followed the ambulance up to the hospital. Then Lys saw them pull the sheet over his head. She did her best to support her mother. Lys had trouble sleeping for a while. She kept dreaming of what happened over and over. Lys also said that all her mother did after Kyle died was sleep.

I called around to see about family counseling. I found out my insurance would cover Lys but not Carley or Noah. I did find one therapist who would take everyone. The rate for Carley and Noah wasn't bad. After talking to me, she brought Lys in separately, then Noah and finally Carley. She spoke to everyone and set up follow up appointments.

On my follow up appointments she told me all of her observations. The doctor said that Lys was fine. Lys didn't view Kyle as a father figure because she had me. As far as her views on Carley and Noah, they were a bit more problematic and worrisome. She said Noah's issues were prominent. He needed more help than she could provide. She couldn't believe Carley was so dismissive. The doctor did her best to talk to Carley about it, but she was very defensive. The doctor said Carley was probably suffering from depression, but she didn't want help. There was nothing the doctor could do. After the follow-up appointment, Carley said she wouldn't go again.

I knew I wanted to file for full custody. I still wasn't sure if that was the right way to go. First off, I didn't have the money to do it. There were ways to do it without hiring an attorney. I would need Lys to say she wanted to live with me. I talked to Lys about everything. She refused even to consider it. She said she needed to go back to take care of her mom.

The counselor had mentioned this. She was worried that Lys was trying to mother Carley instead of the other way around. Lys just needed to be a kid. Right now, Lys was dealing with more adult things than she should have had to. My best option was to keep things how they were. I would have to keep an annoying close eye on everything. I made sure to send more money with Lys than I had been. I also told her if they needed food or something to let me know. I would do what I had to. I talked to Carley's neighbor, and she assured me she would keep an eye on things. The good thing was I was a full-time dad, and Lys knew I was available 100% of the time.

To the surprise of no one, Carley moved her boyfriend Joel in less than two weeks after Kyle had died. Part of me was shocked that it took her that long. I believe Carley was dating Joel a long time before Kyle died. Lys had talked to me about him a few times. Lys told me about a fight Kyle had with Carley a few weeks before he died. Kyle came home from work to find Joel inside the house. He threw Joel out and told Carley he didn't want Joel in the house again. When Carley moved Joel in, it was upsetting to Lys.

Lys asked why her mother would move Joel in knowing Kyle didn't want him in the house. I was shocked by the story and yet not all that surprised. I didn't have an answer for Lys. I told Lys she would have to ask her mother. I also knew from Kyle's family that they would not be giving Carley a dime because she moved someone in. I asked Carley what she was going to do. She said she was going to go back to school. I did not understand how she could even consider that. She needed an income. I asked her what she planned to do for money. She said Joel was going to pay everything. I didn't bother arguing with her. I did feel bad for Joel, and I didn't even know him.

I was starting to get worried because Lys's freshman year was a mess. She was struggling with everything. I think it had a lot to do with all the chaos at her mother's house. I knew something was up. She had gone from an A-B student to flunking a few classes. This wasn't who she was. She was taking her pills, so I knew that wasn't it. Lys said there was a lot of fighting going on at Carley's house. Lys said that Joel was jealous and obsessive. Lys would get woken up by fighting. She would just pull the covers over her head at times.

I asked Lys if she wanted to live with me, and she said no. I was frustrated because Lys wasn't making decisions that were best for her. Lys was still doing what was best for her mom. I was mad at Carley for not letting Lys be a kid. I talked to Lys about forcing the issue, and she still begged me not to. I did get the feeling that she wasn't as steadfast as she had been in the past.

At the end of her freshman year, Lys came to me and asked if she could try out for cheer. She wanted to do it. Now that I was retired, we had the time to do it. With golf, cheer, and softball, her schedule was going to be packed. I warned her how busy she was going to be, but she didn't care. She was thrilled and excited. I was proud of her for wanting to stay active. I did tell her she would have to get her grades back up. I told her if she didn't, then I would make her quit. Her current grades and effort were not nearly good enough. She would have to buckle down. Lys promised me she would work harder.

Her summer was just insane! Lys had golf one day a week. She had softball 2-3 days a week, and she had cheer three days a week. We would go from one thing to another several times. One reason Lys loved to stay so busy is it kept her out of her mother's house. During the summer I saw her almost every day. I think it was essential she knew I was around.

Carley started fighting with Lys about telling me things. She told her not to tell me anything. But Lys is brilliant. She found a way around that. For example, she may post on Facebook, something like I could use some chicken nuggets and fries right now. What that meant was I am hungry, and we don't have food. I would get her food and take it to her. It wasn't always for food. We also had codes for when no one was there, or when Lys didn't feel safe. We had codes for just about everything that could go on.

We decided to take one more vacation while we could. Lys would soon be taking advanced classes in high school. That would make it almost impossible to get away. On this trip, we wanted to go to Universal Studious and Sea World. Lys and I both looked through everything and picked a hotel. The hotel we chose seemed to check all the boxes I had. They had an onsite restaurant and a food court area. They offered transportation to any amusement park. They even had an onsite water park.

I called the hotel personally and asked about their wheelchair, accessible rooms. They said they did have accessible rooms with fully equipped bathrooms with roll-in showers. They told me they had a bus with a lift on it. I would have to reserve that a day ahead. They also had a huge arcade and a movie theater that showed short 4D movies. The whole hotel just seemed terrific.

The first problem of the trip came when we got to the room. We tried to get through the door, and there was a considerable step of about 6-8 inches high. It wasn't easy to get over, but we did it. We got the luggage in and looked around the room. I went into the bathroom. I was not happy at all with what I found. All the shower controls were way out of reach for anyone in a wheelchair. I tried to use the bathroom. I realized two more issues. First, the towel racks that were just above the handrails. They stuck out about 6 inches further than the handrails, so when I stood up to go to the bathroom, I whacked myself in the head with the towel rack and almost fell over. The toilet wasn't the right height either.

I went up to the front desk to see if they had any other rooms that were wheelchair accessible. I talked to the manager who claimed to be part owner. His name was Mohamad; he reminded me of Percy. He was arrogant and cocky and acted like the rules didn't apply to him. I explained that I had just checked in, and I had a few issues. He said that all his handicapped were the same. He told me I was free to find another hotel, but I had prepaid for the week, and it was nonrefundable. I would have to do my best to work around the issues. I asked about the wheelchair accessible bus. They said I could book it for the next morning. I told them we planned on going to Sea World. They told me about the departure time.

We spent the rest of the day at the waterpark and had fun. Lys was having a blast playing with the other kids. The water park had a huge bucket that filled up with water and dumped every few minutes. Once a day, the giant bucket dumped green slime. Soon a loud alarm went off to alert everyone; it was slime time. The bucket tipped over. Green fluid poured all over the awaiting kids below.

After dinner, we decided to check out the 4D movies. We thought the unlimited bands would be the way to go. We realized stairs were leading to the movie theater. We could not find a wheelchair accessible entrance. We went back to where we bought the tickets and asked them. They said they had a hidden elevator. The worker came over and unlocked a small door to reveal a very tiny lift that they installed in a broom closet. I wasn't sure if my chair would fit.

According to the worker, a lot of people had the same issue. He suggested that we go down to the exit of the theater. He would open the door and let us in. I could sit at the bottom and watch the movie from the front. The problem was I did not get any of the 4D effects sitting there. I went and had another chat with Mohammad. He refused to give me any money back. He said he is aware that the elevator is too small, but that wasn't his problem. He said it was my fault for not making sure I could get into the theater before I bought the wristbands.

I tried my best to put aside my issues with the hotel and focus on the rest of the trip. Lys is an animal lover; she was excited about Sea World. We were all loaded on the bus, and everything seemed fine. The bus driver could not get the lift to fold back up. It wouldn't close all the way. The driver had no clue what was going on. Finally, a mechanic arrived from the bus company and got it figured out. We made it to Sea World two hours later than expected. We had to push it to get everything in.

They have a game area with carnival games. Lys loves doing stuff like this. She asked if she could play a couple of games. Lys wanted to play this ring toss game. She threw one, and it bounced off the bottle, flipped up in the air, and landed perfectly on top of the bottle. The guy running the game was shocked! Lys was so happy. She got to pick a prize from the big stuffed animals. She chose this huge black and purple fish. She instantly named him Fishy. The guy said we could leave our name and pick it up at security when we left for the day. I said, OK. I didn't want to carry it all day. Lys, however, wanted no part of that. She was afraid they would lose Fishy.

Let me describe Fishy. He was about 3 foot long and about 2 foot wide at his head. I tried to explain to Lys that it would be complicated to lug it around all day. Lys insisted, so we now were a party of 3. I already hated this damn fish. Everywhere we went, Fishy would get his own spot. Several people asked where we got him. A worker in one of the souvenir shops was very jealous. She had been trying to win one for months. She offered to buy him. I entered into some negotiations only to get yelled at by Lys.

Fishy even got to go with us to a special surprise I had arranged. Lys loves penguins, and I paid extra so we could pet a penguin. I called ahead to make sure it was wheelchair accessible. They said only parts of the tour were. They would figure something out and make sure it was awesome. When Lys found out, she was excited.

Eventually, it was time to head over to the penguin area for our tour. They explained that they didn't have a way to get me up the stairs. We were ushered to a back hallway and told someone would be right with us. Soon a lady walked up to us and introduced herself as one of the head penguin trainers. It was her job to take care of them and make sure they were healthy. The trainer would be spending some time with us and answer any questions we had. She would also be bringing out a penguin in a few minutes. We would get to spend some time with the penguin.

Soon we were sitting in a hallway with a trainer and a penguin. She told us all about the different kinds of penguins and how to tell them apart. She let us feel his feet and flippers. We got to pet him! Then she went to get a different type of penguin. The trainer was walking down the hallway, and a penguin was walking in front of her. As he walked by offices, he would turn his head and look inside. It was cool to see. I think we got to spend about 30 minutes with the trainer and two penguins. We ended up having something even more special than the regular tour.

After dinner, we had to start heading to the bus. I was a bit worried because it appeared to be the same driver. I was praying we wouldn't have any issues. They loaded me on and couldn't get the lift to close up. We were stuck again. We sat for about an hour. Another hour passed and the company sent another bus, but it didn't have a lift.

The driver said help was on the way and should be there soon. Another hour passed before a wheelchair bus showed up. We were able to unload and get headed back to the hotel. The total time we had spent on the bus was about 5 hours. When we finally got back to the hotel, I went right up to the front desk. I looked at the clerk and told her to get me the manager on duty. The clerk said we would have to talk to Mohammad in the morning. I had little hope he would do a damn thing. I was worried that we would not even have transportation to Universal Studios.

Mohammad was looking for us when we went to the front desk. He ran straight over and shook my hand like we were old friends. I was a little shocked. We both knew Mohammad had been fighting with me for days. I wasn't buying his newfound friendship. I knew he would say and do anything to save his ass. I knew he would lie if he thought it was his best for him to do so. Mohammad apologized for all the complications we have had since we had been there. He said he felt horrible about the issues with the bus. He told me the bus was broke.

Mohammad calmed my fears and said he had a plan. He took us outside to where there was a row of taxis and chauffeur driven cars. He motioned for one of them to come over. He introduced us to the driver named Amir. He told us that Amir would be our private driver for the rest of our stay. Mohammad said Amir would take us anywhere at any time we wanted to go. He would just submit the bill to the hotel. I still didn't trust him. I said OK and then told Amir we wanted to go to Universal. Amir gave me his card and told me to call him about 30 minutes before we wanted him to pick us up. When we were walking to the park, I saw a sign that advertised the comedy show Blue Man Group. I asked Lys if she wanted to go. I knew they were funny, and I could use some laughs.

When we entered the park, Lys wanted to get a map and plan where we would go first. I told her all I cared about was getting back to the Harry Potter area. The first thing I saw was the engine for the Hogwarts Express, and it was cool. Then we went through all the shops. The shops were neat but small and hard to get a wheelchair around. I did buy some chocolate frogs and other candy.

We both got wands that chose us. I wanted one of the robes, but Lys said no on multiple occasions. Lys said they were too expensive. I found it funny she was telling me something was too expensive. I know damn well the real reason she wouldn't let me get one. Lys knew I would wear it. I was still disappointed she wouldn't let me geek all out. We tried butter beer, and it was delicious. It is basically like a butterscotch root beer.

Once we left the Harry Potter area, we walked around and rode all the different rides. Before we knew it, we had just enough time to eat before Blue Man Group. The show was even better than I expected. We laughed nonstop and had a blast. I think Lys loved it more than I did. She wanted a program to get autographs from the cast. Lys was so excited to meet them. It was worth every penny for the show. We had had a rough few days, and the laughs helped put me in a much better frame of mind.

Before we could fly home, I had one problem. I had no clue how I was going to get Fishy home. He was way too big to take as a carry-on. When I suggested leaving him at the hotel, Lys got upset. I called the airline to see if there was anything they could do. Fishy would be considered oversized baggage. He would cost me about $35 to get home. They put him in a huge plastic bag with a claim sticker on him. I called my mom to tell her our flight was on time and to tell her how many bags we had. I told her the story of Fishy, and all she could do was laugh. She said that sounded like something Lys would do.

Chapter 20

When we got home, Lys started talking about her mother kicking Joel out. Carley was saying she had enough of him. I was sure she had found someone else. I waited a few weeks, and Carley called me to tell me what was going on. She said the new guys' name was Jaxson. Carley said to me that he had a great job and made a lot of money. She said that he didn't want her to work and she would be able to stay home. Seriously by this point, I was trying hard not to laugh. I knew Carley was just trying to blow smoke up my ass.

I knew Carley was going to do whatever she wanted. I tried to stay focused on the essential things like planning a birthday party for Lys. She wanted a bowling party for her birthday. The highlight of the party was it was going to be the first time I would meet Jaxson. When I met Jaxson, he was what I expected. He looked like a white trash guy who hung out in smoke-filled bars. I got a creepy vibe from him. I was worried about Lys now. I couldn't put my finger on it, but something about him wasn't right. I tried just to blow it off, but it wasn't working.

We were having a good time. Jaxson decided he wanted to talk to me. He kept saying we are going to make sure Lys doesn't date losers, and we will protect her. When Jaxson said we he meant him and I. Which would have been strange on any level, but I had just met this guy. I needed to make it clear that we weren't doing shit. I didn't say any of that to him yet. I knew Carley, and I would be having a serious chat. The more Jaxson talked, the more he creeped me out. I finally gave Carley the death stare. She realized she better get him away from me.

Outside of the mess with Jaxson and Carley, we did get some good news. Lys got accepted into the Skill Center class she wanted. She would be taking courses for veterinarian medicine. Lys is a true animal lover and always wanted to work with animals. She was so excited about school. We went to an orientation to hear about what the class entailed. The teacher showed the book for the course, and it was the size of a giant Webster's dictionary. I admit I was worried for Lys. She had Trigonometry and a few other college prep classes. She would have to work hard this year. I had faith in her, but I knew it was a lot on her plate.

Just as the school year started, I got another surprise. Carley told me she had a job. She wanted me to pick Lys up from school and drop her off at her house. She even offered me gas money. I doubted I would ever see it. I said I would pick Lys up, but I would bring her back to my place. That way, she could get any homework done and I would make dinner. I said if Carley wanted to, she could pick Lys up after work. If she didn't, I would just take Lys to school the next day. Carley wasn't happy about it, but I didn't care.

The more time Lys spent with me, the more she would talk about things. Lys said Carley and Jaxson would fight all the time. Lys spoke about how Jaxson drank beer all day. He would be gone for long periods and then come home drunk. Lys also said that Jaxson and Noah had gotten into a few physical fights. It was clear this was not a good situation, and it was getting worse. I asked Lys again about just living with me. For the first time, she didn't say no. She said she would have to think about it. That told me all I needed to know.

Carley called me and said she had a different job. She said that the new job would be a third shift. Carley wouldn't be able to keep Lys and get her to school. Lys would have to stay with me during the week. Carley tried to get me to let her have Lys every weekend. I laughed at her and told her no. I did agree on every other weekend, but that was all she was getting.

I wasn't happy about paying child support, seeing I had Lys full time. Carley agreed she said she would give it back. I should have gotten something in writing. I knew Lys would be safe and away from all the chaos. I talked to Lys about everything. In typical Lys fashion, she was unfazed by the changes. Lys acted like she didn't care at all. This would be a change for both of us. I was happy and excited about having my baby all the time.

At first, it was strange because we always had the same schedule. Sundays were cleaning and laundry. I always seemed to be in a time crunch between cleaning and making dinner. I can remember the first few weeks I would be stressing about time. Then it would dawn on me that we had all the time in the world. We settled into a new routine reasonably quickly. My body got used to having a week where I could sleep in and get my energy back. Now I was plowing through 12 out of 14 days. Add to that the fact that softball had started workouts. While it may seem like I am complaining, I am not. I loved it, and I loved having Lys all the time. I was just tired. But it was a good tired!

Lys seemed happy and was enjoying being with me full time. She had gone to her mother's one weekend. She said it was strange only being there for two days. I asked her how her mother liked her new job, and she said that Carley quit after the first week. I was shocked! Not that she had quit her job. I had known she didn't want to work. But because Carley did not attempt to ask if we could go back to our actual custody arrangement.

I called Carley to see what was going on. I had a feeling she was going to try and surprise me. Carley explained why she quit. Carley also said she was going to get a different job soon. She mentioned wanting to take Lys for a week. The week Carley wanted Lys just happened to be spring break. I had plans for us that week. I wasn't going just to let Carley do what she wanted. If she wished to have Lys the following week, then she could. I rattled off her schedule, and Carley didn't seem thrilled. She did ask if she could have Lys on Easter. I said yes, because my family didn't have any plans.

Just before spring break, Lys asked if one of her friends Starr could spend the weekend. I told her she could. I always loved it when Lys had friends over. I tried and have an open-door policy, especially when one of her friends needed a place to stay. Starr would come home with Lys on Friday and stay till Sunday. I picked up Lys from school that day, and Starr followed. My first impression of Starr was that she was a cute tiny little thing. I could also tell Starr was very shy. I tried talking to her, and she didn't say a word.

I took them to a store and told them they could get any snacks they wanted. They came out about 30 minutes later with more snacks then you would think two small girls could eat. Once we got home, they went into Lys's room. I could hear them talking and laughing occasionally. I love hearing Lys and her friends laugh together.

The next morning Starr talked to me a little. I knew it was a big step for her. I could tell that her home life wasn't that great. She just looked like a kid who needed someone she could trust. My heart went out to her. I would do what I could for her. Before I knew it, the weekend was over, and Starr was going home. She said I was different than her other friend's dads because I didn't seem to yell. I just laughed and told her I didn't like to yell. I told her she could come over anytime she wanted to.

The next time I would see Starr would be over spring break. I knew this would be the best chance to go prom dress shopping. This was not the first time I had taken Lys dress shopping. I enjoyed being the kind of dad that would do it. We made plans to go to an outlet mall. Lys wanted some friends to go with us. One would be Starr, and the other would be Cheyenne. It would be a long weekend, but I knew the girls would have fun. We decided to go dress shopping first. I quickly realized that we made a huge mistake by going on a Saturday. The store was more than packed.

I had given Lys a budget. I knew I would pay more if she wanted a particular dress. Typically prom dresses are longer, but Lys was never normal. She wanted a shorter one because it would be easier to dance in. Lys found one dress on a mannequin. She loved it, but she couldn't find it in the store. The girls were talking. They were trying to formulate a plan to take it off the mannequin without getting into trouble. I thought they were joking, but they were dead serious.

I convinced them to search the store first. We all took a section of the store to find it. I was able to find the dress Lys wanted in a rack near the back of the store. There was a long line for the changing rooms. They tried to find a few more dresses to try on. So we came up with a plan. They parked me in the changing room line. I would move up with it. They would load me up with dresses to try on. Then I texted them when I got close to the front.

I started looking around, and I realized I was the only man in this entire store. You really would be shocked how many times I would go with Lys and am the only man. I ended up with six dresses on my lap while trying to keep pace with the line. The girls ran up and grabbed the dresses, and headed off to the changing room.

First, Lys tried on the dress I found. The dress fit her perfectly, and she was in love with it. I knew from the smile on her face that we had a winner. Starr came out wearing a short blue sparkly dress that was Lys's second choice. I knew Starr didn't have a prom dress. Lys asked if I would buy it for Starr. I said, sure no problem. I ended up spending less than the budget I had given Lys. Thankfully Cheyenne already had her dress because I wasn't going to buy three.

The next week was Easter, and Carley picked Lys up. They were going to Jaxson's family's house. I got the feeling Lys wasn't thrilled with the idea. I figured she would be gone all day. I was shocked when she was home a few hours later. I could tell something was wrong when Lys walked in. She was upset. I had never really seen her like this. I didn't press her to talk. I figured if she wanted to speak, she would. I knew if I pushed her too hard or too soon, she would shut down. About an hour after she got home, she came into the living room. She sat on the couch, staring into space.

I could tell she just needed a nudge to talk. I asked her if she had fun. All I got was a huge sigh. Lys started to cry. Then she asked if she didn't want to go back to her mother's did she have to? I said absolutely not. I explained to Lys that she would never have to go back if she didn't want to. I asked Lys what happened. She said that Jaxson had started drinking. He and Noah got into a verbal argument. Then Jaxson started punching him. Lys went on to tell me this wasn't the first time. Lys said he never got violent with her, but he had with Noah. Lys told me that Noah had moved in with an aunt weeks before. Lys couldn't understand why her mother would stay with someone like that. I hugged her and told her it would be OK.

I told Lys that she would have to be the one to tell her mother. I told her if it came from me, Carley would think I put Lys up to it. Lys had agreed, and she understood she had to do it. I hated that she was in this situation. Lys was old enough now that she had to deal with it. I would be there for her as much as I could. I knew the talk with Carley had to be just them. That way, Lys could say what she had to from her heart. I don't think all of this is from Easter. I believe that Easter was just the tipping point. Living with me allowed Lys to be a kid without all the drama.

A few days later, after practice, I drove Lys over to her mother's house so they could talk. Lys was nervous. She didn't want to hurt her mother. Lys knew she had to do this. Lys was there for about 45 minutes. I could tell she had been crying. I asked her if she was OK, and she shook her head, yes. I left it at that, and we went for ice cream. Lys said that her mother was upset but didn't fight with her. Carley told Lys that she was going to break up with Jaxson. I was very proud of Lys. She had a lot of guts and internal strength to go against her mother. I hoped that this would be the end of all of the drama. I knew better than to think it was over.

I called Carley a few days later to inform her I was going to cancel child support. I knew the news wouldn't go over well. She started yelling at me, saying that was her money. Carley said that if I tried to cancel the child support, she would fight me. She would force Lys to stay there for a week even though Lys didn't want to. This put me in a tight spot. For the sake of Lys and to not put her through any unneeded drama, I agreed to keep paying.

As Lys's junior year wrapped up, we found out she got accepted to the 2nd year of the veterinarian medicine class. She was so excited. I had already booked an appointment for her senior pictures. We had started looking for driver's education classes to get that done. There was one last year of softball and cheer. This year was going to be crazy! I knew after everything was said and done that I would miss all the practices and games.

Carley's birthday was coming up. The original plan was Lys would spend the day with her. I made it clear I didn't want her spending the night around Jaxson. I didn't like him, and I sure as hell didn't trust him. Had it been just Carley, I wouldn't have had an issue. She was still living with Jaxson. I got a phone call from Carley saying that Lys was going to be spending the night. Carley said they had asked Lys and she wanted to. I was furious! I don't doubt Lys had said yes. She was already there and surrounded by them. What in the hell was she supposed to say?

I started going off about everything that had happened. I told Carley I knew what happened at Easter and that Jaxson had attacked Noah. Carley said to me Noah was there and that he had apologized for starting it. I was furious now. It made no damn sense that Noah should apologize to Jaxson. What kind of mother doesn't support her child? She screamed at me, and I yelled at her. We had the biggest fight we have had in a long time. We fought for at least 30 minutes. I finally hung up on her.

I texted Lys most of the night to make sure she was OK. Lys said that her mother did try to talk her into staying all week. I had spoken to Noah not long after this. He and Jaxson got into another fight. Instead of hitting him, he took Noah's laptop and destroyed it. I felt terrible for him. He had a nice laptop until Jaxson broke it. Yet again, Carley did nothing about it. She said Jaxson would buy Noah a new laptop, but I don't know if he did.

The final straw was a few weeks later. Lys got a phone call from her friend Harleigh. Harleigh said she and Jaxson were talking online. Jaxson started hitting on her and making sexual advances on her. Harleigh was only 17, and Jaxson knew that. Her family went to the police with all the screenshots and filed a report. The police said there wasn't anything they could do because Harleigh was 17. I thought 17 was still considered a minor. They said no, not in that case. We told Carley what had happened, and she was mad. She said she wanted to break up with Jaxson. She may have said that, but she lived there for a few more months.

A few weeks after the blow-up, we had senior pictures taken. I had a hard time believing that my baby was a senior. My first call was to my friend Amber who has a photography studio. I called her, and she was more than happy to do the pictures. I did ask her about hair and makeup. I wanted them done professionally. I was hoping she knew someone. Amber said she knew people that would do it. I also asked her for a favor. I knew with Starr's situation, and she wouldn't get senior pictures done. I wanted her to have the full senior experience. Plus, Lys wanted some best friend pictures.

I explained to Amber the situation. She was more than happy to help me out for a minimal additional cost. Finally, it was picture day, and the girls were over the moon, excited. We had some inside pictures and pictures in a local flower garden. Once I saw the proofs, I was amazed! Amber did such a fantastic job. I remember the first one I saw was Lys in her prom dress, sitting in a flower garden. She looked like a model. They were breathtaking, and the girls loved them so much. Every picture was just perfect.

Once pictures were done, I took both of the girls' school shopping. I made sure Starr had school supplies, a couple of outfits, and some boots she loved. I wanted to make sure Starr started her senior year on the right foot. The more she trusted me, the more she would open up. I had told her she could live with us. I really wasn't sure how I would have afforded it. I would have found a way. She said the reason she didn't move in with us was that our apartment was small. I think part of it was I had warned her if she moved in, she would have to live by the same rules. She knew I was strict, and she had never had a lot of rules.

Senior year for Lys was going to be busy. For part of the veterinary medicine class, Lys would be job shadowing. She would have to job shadow for 12 hours a week for eight weeks. I came up with a plan. I had to get the school to agree with it. Lys had her first hour from 8-9 am every day. Then two online classes at school. I wanted the school to let her miss the online courses for eight weeks. Lys would just do the work at home.

Thankfully the school said the plan worked for them. What I did was drop Lys off to her first hour and wait for her. We would then race off to the job shadowing. Then we would either go home or head to drivers education. I would do whatever I had to for her. I wasn't looking for any kind of award. I was just proud that I had a daughter who knew what she wanted to do. She was following her heart and willing to work hard to make her dreams come true.

I knew we needed to start figuring out what college Lys would be attending. I thought Lys would go to Mott as I did. The plan I had was for her to go there for two years and get a base degree. Then transfer somewhere with a veterinarian program. Lys mentioned that another local college named Baker had talked to her at skill center about their vet program. We set up an appointment to go and speak to them.

I was impressed by what Baker had to say. If Lys went there, she could get an Associate's degree as a veterinarian technician. They gave us a full tour of the facilities. They talked at length about the cost. This school was more expensive then Mott. Thankfully Lys would qualify for financial aid. They would also help with student loans. Lys was ready to start right then. We talked on the way home. We both agreed it was perfect.

Now that we had college all set, we could focus on the rest of Lys's senior year. I was already getting sad that taking Lys to games and practices was coming to an end. I knew I would miss it. Some of our best talks about life had been traveling to and from games. We talked about what happened in the game and life lessons you can take from it. I know every sports parent goes through the same issues. I wouldn't trade all those memories for anything.

I made sure to go to every game. Some of the schools we played were in the middle of nowhere. Thankfully I had gotten a power wheelchair. I would never have made it in a regular wheelchair. I loved watching Lys play. As the season went on, the end got closer. I started to dread each game. Softball was such a big part of our lives. I never wanted it to end. Eventually, it did end. On senior day I cried. I was sadder about softball ending than I was about Lys graduating high school.

Leading up to Lys's graduation and graduation party, I knew I was facing a real problem. The problem was the party was at my sister's house. My mom did not want any of Carley's side of the family invited. To be honest, she didn't even want Carley invited. There was some serious bad blood between everyone. Lys wanted both sides of the family to be there.

I fought with my mom and sister for several days before they finally gave up. Part of the sales pitch was I could get Carley's family to help. I knew I couldn't trust Carley to get her family organized. So I called her aunt Cindy. I picked Cindy because she was the one who held all the family parties. I knew if there was one person I could trust to get things done, it was her. She went right to work and was a big help. Carley, however, was pissed at me. She was mad; I hadn't called her first. I wish she would have just thanked me. I just explained to her why and told her to get over it.

The events around graduation were a whirlwind. We found out that Lys would graduate with honors. She just missed being part of the top 10 in her class. I was so proud of her. Lys had to deal with a lot, and she never let it stop her. Lys just powered through all of it. There is nothing more satisfying as a parent than to watch your children succeed. Watching Lys walk across the stage and get her diploma was a happy moment for me. It made all the sacrifices worth it. I started to tear up as I watched Lys and Starr graduate. Starr had a lot to be proud of too. Starr told me several members of her family told her she could just quit school because she would never graduate. I gave them both a huge hug and told them how proud I was.

My mom wanted to have Lys's graduation party as soon as possible. We scheduled it for the Sunday after graduation. We couldn't have it on Saturday because we had state playoffs for softball. I felt terrible that we couldn't help set up. The day of the party was hectic. I was worried we wouldn't have a big turnout, but we did. Lys did have a few awkward moments. She didn't know some of the family that was there. A lot of Carley's family was there just how Lys wanted.

The only real drama we had was as we were cleaning up the party. Carley grabbed the card box and presents and tried to put them in her car. I had kind of expected her to try this. I had been keeping a close eye on it. I worried Lys wouldn't get all the money. Carley wanted to make me feel guilty for not trusting her. I made it clear I didn't trust her. I couldn't even believe she was arguing about this. My family heard us fighting and started to walk toward us. Carley gave up and handed me the card box. Lys laughed at her. Lys knew that wasn't going to work. As much as I had anticipated her pulling something, I was still pissed she had tried.

A few months after Lys graduated, I started having health issues again. My doctors believe the issues were, in part, caused by the Flint water crisis. I have a compromised immune system. When I learned about the water crisis, I became concerned. I did all I could to try and not use any tap water. But there were times we had to. The main problem I had was I had an open blister on my foot. My doctor suggested cleaning it real good in a hot shower. I didn't even think about the Flint water when I did it. I went back to the doctor a week later, and my foot was severely infected. My doctor believes that something from the water caused the infection. It got so bad that they thought I might lose my foot.

Thankfully after several months of daily antibiotic IVs, they were able to save my foot. I know some may ask if things are so bad why I haven't moved.

The answer to that question is rather simple; I can't. I have looked, but finding affordable wheelchair accessible housing is very complicated. Especially now that President Trump has changed some of the laws. I do worry about the long term effects the water may have not just on me but Lys as well. I wonder if when she decides to have children, will they be at risk for birth defects. I know the politicians seem to believe it won't be an issue. I don't trust them, and I never will.

Conclusion

First off, I would like to thank everyone who has taken the time to read this book. When I first started writing it, my goal was to try and change people's opinions of people who are disabled. I hope that happens, but I realized I got more out of this than I anticipated. I used to have a great deal of anger and frustration bottled up. As I wrote this book, it forced me to deal with all of it and to be honest. I am much happier because of it. Although I wish some of the things that happened wouldn't have, I wouldn't be who I am without them happening. Too often, we get caught up on all the bad things, and we don't focus on the good things.

I have had far more great things happen in my life than bad. The main reason for that is my mom who pushed me to lead as normal of a life as possible. Even now, she has been there pushing me to finish this book. She remains my biggest supporter. She believed in my story, and without her, this book would not exist. I am thankful that she has managed to beat breast cancer twice and still be here for Lys and me.

As far as Lys and I are concerned, things have been going well for us. We are still dealing with the effects of the Flint water crisis, and I worry about infections every time I take a shower. I have had severe infections now three times that may or may not be water-related. I have wanted to move but, as of yet, have been unable to find suitable affordable wheelchair accessible housing. I have always believed things will happen when they are supposed to, and it will just be a matter of time until I find other housing. The key for me is staying positive and believing that life is a process, and I need to remain patient.

The update for Lys is fantastic. When Lys started college, she did struggle, and she had to retake a few classes. Thankfully Lys battled through it, and she is now just a few months away from graduating with her associates' degree for veterinary technician. I really can't stress enough how proud I am of her. I have seen many of her friends struggle in college and just quit. Lys refused to take the easy way out. This degree is her dream, and she fought for it. She once told me the reason she didn't give up is that she has seen me have to fight every day. Lys said I taught her never to give up. As parents, we never really know how much our children are paying attention. I am glad that if she learned one lesson from me that it was that one.

I know I have learned as much from Lys as she has from me. I used to think that once she turned 18, she wouldn't need me anymore, and my life would mainly be over. Now with completing this book, I realize that I am just getting started. I still have many dreams that I have yet to accomplish, and I will not quit. Much like with Lys in college, I struggled at times to finish this book. I will admit it is far more work than I ever anticipated. I think I made every mistake imaginable on what not to do while writing a book. As usual, though, I have to learn the hard way. The future used to scare me but not anymore.

I am looking forward to new adventures that life will throw at me. Part of that future includes everyone who is reading this book. I hope that you will send me feedback, both positive and negative. Feel free to follow me on Twitter @shortbusworld or Facebook at D.A. Perry. Thanks again for reading, and I love you all!!

CPSIA information can be obtained
at www.ICGtesting.com
Printed in the USA
LVHW040222250920
667092LV00001B/264

9 781632 637697